Recovering Life

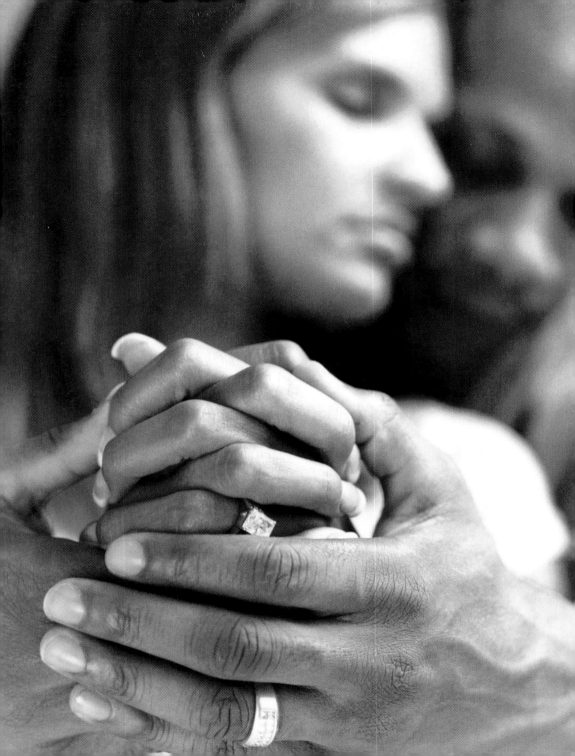

RECOVERING LIFE

CHARISSE & DARRYL STRAWBERRY

THE PLOUGH PUBLISHING HOUSE

Jacket photographs and photographs pp. ii, vi, viii, x, xiv, xviii, 10, 24, 34, 54, 78, 92, 106, 118, 136 copyright © 1999 by Toshi Kazama.

Photographs pp. 8, 26, 32, 53, 117, 138, 140, 142 copyright © 1999 by The Plough Publishing House.

Images pp. 51, 71, 75, 77, 97, 101, 105, 113 courtesy of Charisse and Darryl Strawberry.

Letters pp. 111 and 121-122 reproduced by kind permission of Kirk C. Mackey and Emily Voorhees, respectively.

Text design and production by Mulberry Tree Press & Tania Garcia Design.

First Printing   80,000   November 1999

A catalog record of this book is available from the British Library.

    Library of Congress Cataloging-in-Publication Data

Strawberry, Charisse, 1967-
    Recovering life / Charisse & Darryl Strawberry.
        p. cm.
    ISBN 0-87486-988-9 (hard.)
        1. Strawberry, Darryl—Health. 2. Colon (Anatomy)—Cancer—
Patients—United States—Biography. 3. Baseball players—United
States—Biography. I. Strawberry, Darryl. II. Title.

RC280.C6 S77 1999
796.357'092—dc21
[B]
                                                        99-026740

Printed in the USA.

To Nana, who's been with us through thick and thin.
You're the most strong-willed angel we know —
and a terrific grandmother, great-grandmother,
babysitter, nurse, and cook besides.

To Josh, our guide along the road to recovery.
Your selfless and giving spirit amazes us time and again.
We thank God for the way you lead by example,
and for the courage you give us.

To Eric, who does everything a lawyer and agent could
possibly do for us, and still finds time to be a true friend
and confidant. Thank you for loving us for who we are,
and for watching our backs.

To Ma and Pa Leonard, who've redefined the role
of godparents. Thank you for teaching us that there are two
ways of looking at every situation, and for always reminding
us to keep God first in our marriage and in our lives.

And to all the many people we love, our family and friends
who've supported us and stood side by side with us in our life
together. You were all in our thoughts as we wrote this book,
and we dedicate it to each and every one of you.

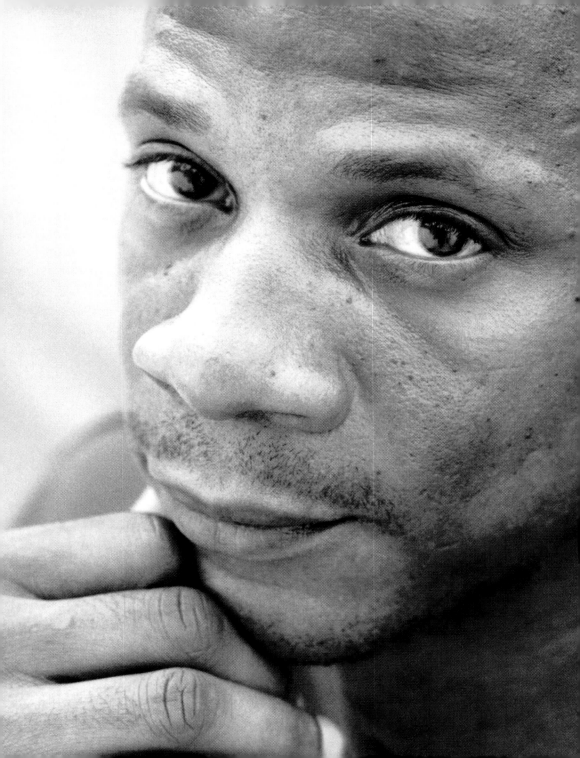

The ultimate measure of a man
is not where he stands in moments
of comfort and convenience,
but where he stands at times
of challenge and controversy.

MARTIN LUTHER KING JR.

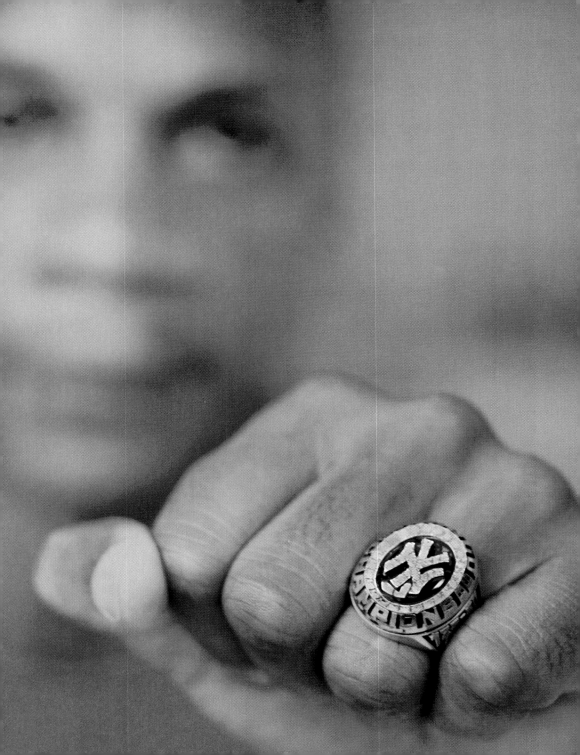

C O N T E N T S

ॐ

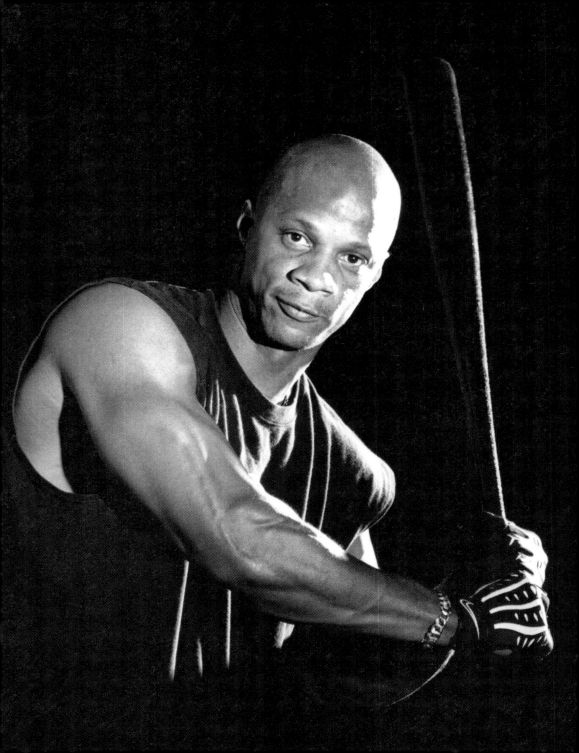

FOREWORD

Since 1996, my rookie year with the Yankees, Darryl Strawberry has been a special part of my life. I see him as a mentor. To me, he's like a big brother who's gone through a lot and wants to protect me. Some people might find that odd, given Darryl's well-publicized failings. But those people don't know him as a person and friend. They don't see Darryl when he's with his wonderful wife, Charisse, and his children. They're not around when he does those quiet things that show you how big his heart really is and how much he thinks about other people and what they're going through.

When I first broke into the big leagues, I had a lot to learn. There's nothing that can prepare you for a career in sports in New York City. You find out quickly how much you depend on the advice of those who have lived under scrutiny for years – on and off the field. There is so much to the game of baseball that only a real pro can teach. Darryl understands a young player's temptations and always has something helpful to say. He is an encourager who quietly and lovingly showed up in my life.

In this book, *Recovering Life*, Darryl and Charisse show the world what it is that keeps them going, even through the hardest times. They reveal a part of their lives that most people have never seen or known about. Through it, I have begun to understand a little bit more about my "big brother."

This is not a book about baseball. It's a book about life, about how to learn from life's experiences, about honesty – with yourself and with those around you. But it happens to be written by a winning team: by a man who has some of the purest baseball talent I've seen, who's able to step to the plate and, with one sweet, breathtaking swing, bring a crowd to its feet; and by the woman who stays right by his side, even when the count isn't in his favor. Thank you, Charisse. And keep swinging, Darryl.

Derek Jeter
Fall 1999

RECOVERING LIFE

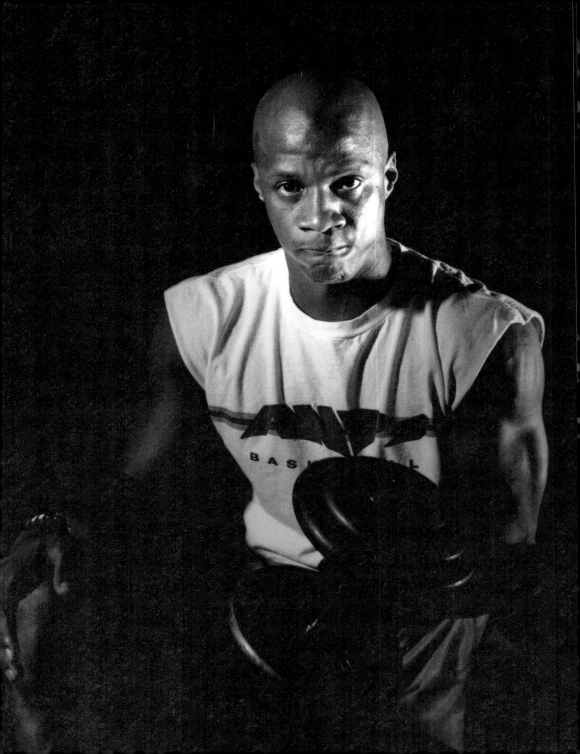

BATTLE STATIONS

As a professional athlete, there's a certain weight you carry everywhere you go. It has to do with expectations. Some people expect good, some bad. On top of that, there are the expectations you place on yourself. Eventually you find yourself lugging a mountain around on your shoulders, but you never really talk about it to anyone. You try to kid yourself that this is "normal," and so you never really get around to dealing with your feelings. At least not until something comes along and slaps you across the face and forces you to stop in your tracks and pay attention – something like cancer.

My battle against cancer began in October 1998 – or at least that's when I started fighting back. Since then, it's changed everything: nothing can be taken for granted anymore. It's changed the way Charisse and I feel and think, how we view the world and the people around us, our perspectives on our own lives and our children's lives.

Shortly after Darryl heard that he had cancer, someone asked him whether he thought it was "fair" that he of all people was going to have to face this disease. I'll never forget Darryl's response: "Well, why not me..."

I'm sure he wasn't trying to be profound at the time, but by saying that, Darryl summed up the way he and I want to approach everything we're confronted with in life. There are no guarantees – anything can happen to anyone at any time – so why get caught up in questioning the "fairness" of life?

Over the years we've been together, we've learned a lot about what it means to trust in God's plan. It's not always easy, but we do our best to help each other remember that, no matter what happens, our lives are in his hands.

Darryl's no angel, and there's no denying the mistakes he's made – or the fact that he's paid dearly for them in both his personal and public lives. Then again, I'm no angel either. None of us is. Some of us are just fortunate enough not to have our shortcomings printed in bold type in newspaper headlines or announced on television.

Darryl and I share the same goal: we want to be the best people we can be, with kindness in our hearts toward everyone. That in itself is a full-time battle, without trying to be perfect on top of it.

So we keep trying, even when we fall short. The most important thing for us, as for anyone, is the attitude we take toward life. It comes down to a very simple question, one we have to ask ourselves every day: are we fighters or quitters?

Cancer brought me up short. It placed me in a battle I'd never bargained for. Once you've been put in that frying pan, well, you realize it's a whole different frying pan from anything you've experienced before. Suddenly you're forced to reevaluate everything, and to think about things you never really took time to consider before. That's what Charisse and I want to talk about in this book: not necessarily so much about cancer (you'll get a sense of what that's like too), but more about the things life has taught us and the lessons we're learning – one day at a time.

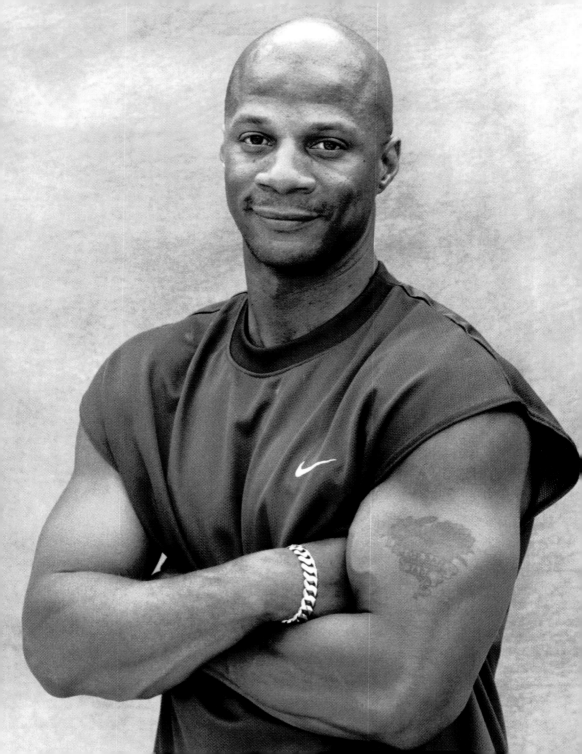

CHAPTER I

WHAT'S NEXT?

"It had to be something more than just
an ulcer or an upset stomach."

– Darryl

"I hadn't really considered the possibility
that Darryl might really be sick."

– Charisse

Looking back, I remember the signs. You know what they say: hindsight is always 20/20. There were times during 1998 when Darryl would complain about stomach pain. There were signs something wasn't right – not necessarily big things, but little changes that developed over the course of the baseball season. His appetite shrank. He'd ask me to fix his favorite recipes for him, then would nibble at his food. I'd get upset: "I'm wasting my time cooking all this food, and you're not eating it…"

There were other changes too. Sometimes I'd wake up at night and he wouldn't be in bed next to me. A light would be on, and he'd be in the bathroom or downstairs in the kitchen, or somewhere. Normally, he sleeps like a baby, so this was unusual. But he'd just shrug it off: "I just can't sleep."

Then Darryl started passing blood, and I got worried. "Go get it checked. You probably have an ulcer." But he'd say, "Nah, it's just hemorrhoids," and I usually let it go at that – he didn't want me fussing over him.

At the time there really didn't seem to be much reason to worry about my husband's health. Whatever was giving him trouble certainly wasn't stopping him on the field. Darryl put up some great numbers, contributing to the Yankees' record-breaking season by hitting 24 home runs and batting in 57 runs in only 295 at-bats.

And then September was as good as over, and it was time for the post-season to begin.

Monday, September 28, was an off-day, the day before we were scheduled to play Game 1 of our Division Championship Series against the Texas Rangers at Yankee Stadium. All of us on the team were looking forward to getting down to business, but we were glad for the day of grace to prepare mentally and emotionally for the series ahead. But as it turned out, by the end of that Monday my thoughts and feelings had little, if anything, to do with baseball. It was an "off-day" in more ways than one.

Don't ask me why I chose that day to talk to Dr. Stuart Hershon, our team doctor. I'd been telling myself for a long time that I needed to get some medical attention, that something inside me wasn't right, but I'm not sure why I went to get checked out the day before our first playoff series opened.

I guess I'd just reached a point where I knew I had to do *something*. Through August and into September the pain in my gut kept intensifying, and now I was having a hard time ignoring it. I wasn't enjoying my meals (and eating is something I love) and I felt lethargic. At night, I was waking up with stomach cramps so painful I'd break into a sweat.

Actually the pain had been there for most of 1998, but if there's one thing you learn as an athlete it's how to suck up pain. A ruptured disc in your spine or a torn knee ligament – those are undeniable injuries because they affect your ability to move. But when your pain is internal, it's easier to keep secret. So I fought between not wanting to admit to myself or Charisse that something was wrong with me, and growing anxiety that this was going on too long. It had to be something more than just an ulcer or an upset stomach. "I need to figure out what's going on," I told myself.

Ten days earlier we had played the Orioles at Baltimore, and while we were there I had sought out my buddy and fellow outfielder Eric Davis (we've known each other since childhood) and told him how I was feeling. In the spring of 1997 Eric had been diagnosed with colon cancer and undergone surgery, and ever since then he'd been preaching early intervention to anyone who'd listen. Now he listened to me describe the pain I was going through and said it reminded him of what he'd experienced before his cancer was discovered. He told me not to mess around, to get it checked out right away.

I made up my mind and saw the doctor.

Darryl didn't tell me he was going to the doctor when he left our home in Fort Lee, New Jersey, that morning. The first I knew of it was when the phone rang and I answered it to hear a doctor from Columbia-Presbyterian Medical Center tell me that Darryl, who had come to see him accompanied by Dr. Hershon, had symptoms of diverticulitis and should go back for more tests.

I don't think I'd ever even heard of diverticulitis before, but it didn't sound like something anybody would want to have. So I started calling up friends, people I knew in the medical field, to pick their brains about it. If something was wrong with my husband, I wanted to know what it was and what I could do to help him through it – and quickly. Neither one of us wanted to see him lose his spot on the playoff roster.

That was Monday. Darryl was in the dugout for Game 1 the next night but wasn't scheduled to play. His chance was supposed to come the following night, Wednesday, in Game 2.

But Wednesday morning we returned to Columbia-Presbyterian for a CAT-scan on Darryl. Obviously the doctors didn't like what they saw, because not long after we arrived back home, the phone rang and Dr. Jonathan LaPook, the gastroenterologist who had overseen the scan, was on the line. The results had revealed a growth on Darryl's colon, he told me, and now they needed to run a colonoscopy to get an inside look. Darryl would have to drink a laxative (Colo-Lyte, I think it was) and clean out his colon, Dr. LaPook explained.

Up until then I hadn't really considered the possibility that Darryl might really be sick. How could he be? Physically, he was in great shape, and right on top of his game. But Dr. LaPook's phone call shook me up. Did the doctors know more than they were letting on? I wondered as I made arrangements to bring Darryl to the hospital early the next morning. Still, I didn't let myself worry all that much. The way the doctors were talking, we'd be flying out of New York later in the day to catch up with the team in Arlington, Texas.

Well, so much for Game 2. We spent the evening at home in front of the TV.

The CAT-scan results didn't sound good, but I was at least glad to know that the doctors were in the process of discovering what was wrong with me, and that my months of trying to second-guess myself would be over. I wanted to get this thing over with and get back to the team. I wanted to be on the field, contributing. Drinking Colo-Lyte and sitting at home weren't high on my list of things to be doing during the playoffs.

Charisse and I went to the hospital Thursday morning. Dr. Hershon and Dr. LaPook met us there. We had to wait a while for another doctor, Dr. George Todd, to show up. He was a surgeon, and Dr. LaPook wanted him present for the colonoscopy.

We waited what seemed like a long time for Dr. Todd to show up. I remember wondering why Dr. LaPook didn't just go ahead with the procedure. Eventually, Dr. Todd showed up.

Darryl was wheeled off to be anesthetized, and I was ushered into another room with a TV screen. When the colonoscopy began, the images from the scope appeared on that monitor. It seemed surreal…

I see the scope travel through Darryl's colon, and everything looks about how you'd expect a colon to look. Then – boom!

The scope reaches a spot that appears red, inflamed, irritated. There I am, watching this by myself, and it's not hard to realize something's definitely wrong with this picture...

Actually, I wasn't exactly alone. Interns came in and out continually, and one of them saw the image on the screen and let out a low whistle. "What?" I asked. But all he would say was, "Your doctor will talk to you about it."

After that, they let me into Darryl's room. He was still very drowsy, more or less out of it. Doctors Hershon and LaPook asked me to sit down. By then I already knew what was coming. "We've found a tumor in Darryl's colon. It's about the size of a walnut," they told me. It was almost completely blocking his colon, they said, which explained his intense pain.

Then they dropped the bombshell.

"... and we think it might be cancerous."

"Cancer?"

I hardly heard the rest of what Dr. LaPook was saying – something about biopsies and more tests and wanting to remove the tumor as soon as possible, and about how curable cancer can be if caught early enough. He had said "cancer," and I guess I just wasn't prepared for that. I mean, who ever heard of a 36-year-old man with cancer? It just wasn't part of my thinking. I started to cry. But only a little, because next we had to tell Darryl, and I wanted to be strong for him...

"So, what's the word?" He's still a bit out of it, but his winner's attitude definitely shines through. "What's up?" he asks again, looking at me. I gulp. "Well, um, Darryl, the doctors say you have a tumor." I refuse to use the word cancer – anyway, it's too soon; they don't know for sure, I tell myself. "It's in your colon," I tell him, "the size of a walnut. They want to take it out right away." I let Dr. LaPook explain the rest. Darryl listens, asks a few questions: mainly he wants to know if he'll be able to recover and play ball again, and the doctors assure him he will…

We talked about the next step. Dr. Todd wanted to schedule surgery for some time the following week, the next Wednesday, I think. Generally it takes several days to get biopsy results, but the doctors promised they'd have them later that night.

I took Darryl home. He lay down for a nap, while I waited for Dr. LaPook's inevitable phone call.

I felt very alone. It was a feeling that kept returning during those first days of uncertainty. But I took comfort in knowing that at any time I could pick up the phone and talk to a friend, someone like Eric Grossman. He's Darryl's agent and our lawyer, but more than that, he's one of the best friends we have, a person who truly cares about us. Eric and I talked many times; just hearing him on the line somehow served to reassure me that everything was going to work out all right.

Darryl was still resting when the phone rang. I picked it up and listened to Dr. LaPook use that word again: cancer. No more maybes or wishful thinking – they were sure about this. He said he had to be in Washington, DC, for the weekend but that he could arrange the surgery for Monday or Tuesday, when he'd be back. I sat there and said to myself, and to God, "Darryl can't wait. We need to get this done now, because we can't sit here for five days with it on our minds."

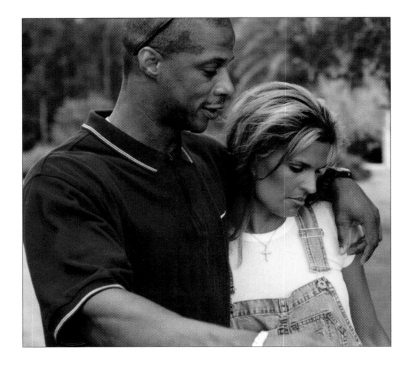

I went upstairs to talk to Darryl. He was lying on the bed and rolled over and looked up at me as I came into the bedroom.

"Well, what are they saying?"

I told him. He sat up.

"So, what's next?"

I didn't really have to ask to know what the doctor had told her. The answer was written all over her face. We sat together on the edge of the bed, and I asked, "What's next?" Not that I meant the question for Charisse – it was more or less my way of trying to grasp what was going on. I mean, what else could happen to me? Right then, I sensed I was facing a mountain tougher than any I'd ever had to climb. Fighting cancer was going to be the biggest fight of my life – literally, a battle against death – and I decided from the start that I was going to give this fight my best effort. I knew that if I was going to have a shot at winning, I couldn't afford to take pity on myself. It was going to be all-out war, and the fight was on. I looked at Charisse and did my best to grin.

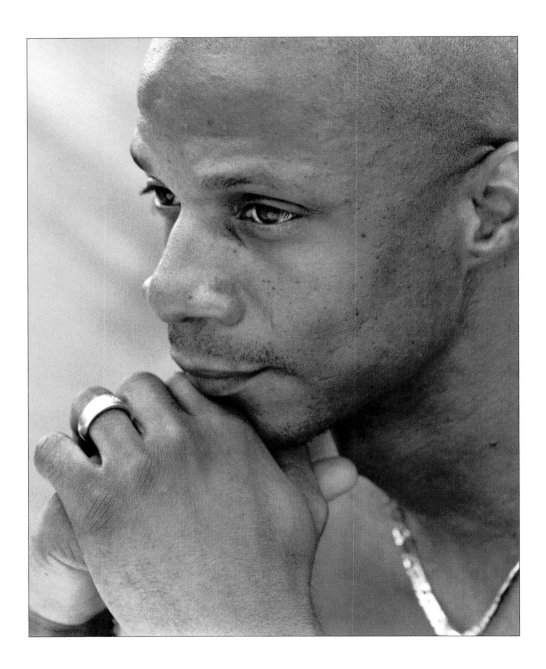

CHAPTER II

LOSING

"No matter what I went through
or what my life was like, Mom always told me,
'I want you to respect other people.'
And you can't put a price tag on that."

"She kept her pain to herself,
hiding it in the pages of her journal."

You could say, I guess, that I came by cancer honestly enough. It runs in our family. I watched it claim my mom's life. She died from breast cancer on February 25, 1996. She had just turned fifty-five on January 29.

My mom, Ruby Strawberry, was the most courageous woman I've ever known. She raised five of us – I have two older brothers, Michael and Ronnie, then there's me, followed by the two girls, Regina and Michelle – and she never once asked anyone for help. She sure didn't get any from my dad. He drank and gambled and kicked all of us around, and then left when I was thirteen. So it was up to Mom and her job as a secretary at Pacific Bell to feed and clothe us. And she did. She saw us all through high school, and stood up for what was best for her kids.

Without a doubt, Mom was hands down the biggest influence I knew in my growing-up years. The most amazing thing about her was, she loved me just for being me. She raised me from the point when there was nothing there, when I was just a handful of cells – long before I was a baseball star.

I was born March 12, 1962, and grew up in Crenshaw, a neighborhood not exactly classed among Los Angeles's finest. It was crowded, with houses right on top of each other, but it wasn't a violent place. People more or less got along with each other. I spent long hours playing football on the street in front of our house, just having a good time. Especially after my dad left and he and Mom divorced, things relaxed around the house and we kids were able to enjoy a little more freedom. Until then my brothers and sisters and I lived in fear of my father and his angry outbursts (I'll talk more about that later). When he left, it gave us our first chance to start discovering who we were, to find out what we wanted to do and explore the things we liked. Mom was a big help. She encouraged each of us to go after our dreams.

My big dream was to become a professional athlete. I penciled a note and stuck it to my bedroom door: "I belong in the majors." I used to fantasize about making it as a big-time baseball player so that I would have a ton of money and could take care of my mom, because even as a kid I knew how hard she worked. I understood that raising five kids on her own was the most difficult part of her life, even though she never let on, and even though my brothers and sisters and I never felt disadvantaged. We always had enough to eat, and clothes and shoes weren't ever a problem.

When it came to other things – bicycles, for example – I learned to be creative. My neighborhood friends and I collected parts from old bikes and put them together, building our versions of "dirt bikes" from them. Then we'd ride the streets around our block, popping wheelies or looking for the biggest curb where we could practice our cross jumps, that kind of thing.

Once I turned thirteen, my life was measured in Saturdays, at least in summer. I lived all week for Saturday morning. That's when I'd get to head for the park and play baseball with my Little League team. I could go out onto the field, and for a while at least, everything else in the world would disappear. All that would be left was just me and baseball.

Believe it or not, once fall came around and the school year started, Monday became my next-best day to Saturday. As much as I looked forward to the weekend, I always was ready to get back to school. A lot of kids in my neighborhood didn't see the point of school, but in my family there was no question about it: you participated in school. My mom understood the importance of education, and she passed that on to us. She didn't put pressure on us about our grades or that kind of thing, but we knew she expected us to give our best effort. Actually, we knew that's what Mom expected of us no matter what we were doing, and you never forget that.

I started high school in 1977, and then athletics really took center stage in my life. In the fall of my junior year, I was the starting quarterback for the football team. That winter I played basketball, and in the spring I started varsity baseball. When Mom saw me play, I guess it kind of shocked her. She'd never seen me show that kind of intensity about anything before. The side of me my mom saw most was the side that sat around the house in a baseball hat eating junk food, the kid who'd rather hang around home with his sisters than run around the streets. When I'd got into Little League at thirteen, she'd come out to my games to cheer me on, but I don't think she thought I took my playing very seriously.

But it wasn't like she was suddenly all impressed with her son, even if everyone said he was going to go far either as a basketball or a baseball player. It wasn't like her to get all puffed up about her children. She was too humble for that. The way she saw it, her job was to love us to death and to make the best life for us out of what she had.

That's something I can't be thankful enough for. You see so many parents of talented teenagers today, and they're pushing their kids to achieve, to make a name for themselves and their families. My mom never did any of that. Even when my major league career got underway, she never got caught up in the hype that followed me around. I was her son, and she loved me for that. That's why it made me so happy finally to be able to fulfill my dream of buying her a beautiful home and seeing her well taken care of, even though she wasn't looking for money or prestige or possessions. She focused her energy on being a person who loved God and her family and stood up for the values she believed in.

More than anyone else in my life, Mom taught me through her example the meaning of respect. She couldn't tolerate big egos. She wanted so much for her children to understand the strength of humility. No matter what I went through or what my life was like, she always told me, "I want you to respect other people." She lived her life by that rule, and she tried to pass it on to her children. You can't put a price tag on that.

God and my mom were close friends. Her faith was what gave her the strength to face motherhood on her own. Without being pushy about it, she encouraged us to find a relationship with God, took us to church with her each Sunday, and told us stories from the Bible. She never said so, but I know it must have hurt her in later years to see me uproot the seeds of faith she'd tried to plant in me. She sure found joy in seeing me reestablish my relationship with God during the last years of her life.

In early 1994, Darryl's mom went to the doctor because of a swollen lymph node under her arm. She had started working out, to get into shape, and perhaps that's what aggravated the node. At any rate, they went in and removed it, and ran a biopsy. It proved to be cancerous, and the doctors recommended she undergo radiation treatment. We took the news pretty hard, but the surgery had gone well and her prognosis was good, which gave us something to be glad about. But one thing about Ruby Strawberry: she always knew what she wanted. She decided against radiation, opting instead for a homeopathic treatment; her fate, she told us, rested ultimately in God's hands, and she was happy to leave him in charge of her future.

For the better part of that year Darryl's mom seemed to be doing okay. Then in December she had more pain in her arm, and she agreed to start chemotherapy. Meanwhile, Darryl and I were on the move again. By April 1995 the baseball strike, which had cut short the 1994 season, was over. Darryl finished serving his suspension and signed with the Yankees. In June we headed for Tampa, Florida, where Darryl trained for a while before joining the Triple-A team in Columbus; it would be midsummer before he finally got to New York. When we left California and our desert home in Rancho Mirage (near Palm Springs), his mother seemed in surprisingly good health as we said our good-byes.

What we didn't know was that already then she was heading downhill. After we arrived in New York, she started losing ground – the cancer was spreading, and she decided to quit treatment. But we didn't know it, and neither did any of her other children. So when we got back to California in October 1995, after the Yankees' post-season loss to Seattle, we were in for a shock. We hardly recognized her, she looked so different. She had lost her hair as a result of the chemotherapy. From then on she wore a wig, which actually looked quite cute on her. But it was as if the cancer was sucking the life right out of her, she was so worn out.

And then, right after our return, as we watched the condition of Darryl's mom grow worse, Bill Goodstein, Darryl's agent, died unexpectedly of a heart attack. We were devastated. He died when we needed him most, and that was one of the saddest days we've known. We were dealing with a lot of issues at that time, including renegotiating Darryl's contract with the Yankees, and Bill was the guy who took care of everything for us. We knew he had diabetes and poor circulation – at one point there was even talk of amputating his legs – but still we never expected to lose him without warning. He was only in his fifties.

I was the last person to talk to Bill. He called me at our home in Rancho Mirage from his office in New York on Saturday morning, January 13th, and I answered the phone to his usual greeting, "Hey, kid-o," and we chatted a while. Sunday morning, his son-in-law Eric Grossman called me as I was driving to church with Jordan and Jade. He was crying. "Charisse, I've got bad news."

"What happened?" I'd never heard Eric so distressed before. He told me that after I'd got off the phone with Bill the day before, he'd had a heart attack and died in his office on Madison Avenue.

I didn't want to believe it. I mean, Bill was just the best guy, one of the best friends we'd ever had.

Bill was like an angel sent to us by God; he came out of nowhere at a time when I was in need of an agent with a head on his shoulders to represent me. It was early 1995, and my days on the West Coast were up. A friend recommended we talk with Bill, and that was the beginning of a wonderful friendship, one that ended much too soon.

Bill became my agent in the spring of 1995, and that summer he got me my first contract with the Yankees. He knew I belonged in New York. He'd say, "This town loves you, Darryl, no matter what happens to you. How can they ever forget what you did for the Mets, the years you had over there? You *belong* in New York," like he was a preacher or something. He could be so funny when he got on his soapbox, and he'd go on and on like that. He wasn't afraid to take his message to George Steinbrenner (he owns the Yankees) and tell him just exactly why I belonged on the team.

After meeting me for the first time, Bill told his son-in-law, "Eric, you're not going to believe this. You wouldn't even know Darryl's a baseball player, because he doesn't act like one."

On top of being a well-respected lawyer, Bill understood the business side of sports, especially baseball, and had represented several high-profile athletes in the past. But he was more than just a heads-up agent. In a world where so many people wanted to be around me because of who I was or what they thought I could offer them, Bill was someone I could trust. He wasn't after money; that just wasn't his game. Friends like that are invaluable.

It was almost like he adopted Charisse and me as his kids. He and his wife, Barbara, had two daughters, Lauren and Cindy, and they were all very close, but Bill had room for us as well. We were like family to him.

In 1995, when we moved to New York and lived in West-chester, I used to go into the city with my kids and "Nana" (my dad's mother) when Darryl was on the road, and we'd go over to Bill's office, just to sit there. I was scared to death in New York City. Once, my grandmother talked me into taking the train, but it unnerved me, and I swore "never again" after that. So we'd hang out in Bill's office, which could have been straight out of the set for a baseball movie, there was so much memorabilia everywhere. Bill and I became really close friends, and we talked all the time. I think I spent more time on the phone with him than Darryl did, because Darryl was always away playing or something.

Darryl was already at church when Eric called me on my car phone to say Bill had died, and my eyes were so full of tears I could barely see the road. I just kept saying to myself, over and over, "Oh, my God." I was crying and crying, and I had to pull Darryl out of church and tell him. Then we went back in and sat down, each of us trying to comfort the other. At the end of the service, we asked for prayers, both for us and for the Goodstein family.

We flew to New York from Los Angeles for Bill's funeral. That's where we met Barbara for the first time – at her husband's funeral. It made me realize how we'd never really seen Bill in his home environment. She took my face in her hands and said, "Oh, you're as lovely as Bill said you were." And she hugged Darryl and told him, "Bill loved you guys so much." We were all crying. And then we all drove out to Long Island through the falling snow, for the burial. After the casket was lowered, we each picked up a handful of dirt and threw it down into the grave.

I cried so hard at Bill's funeral service. Even after everybody left, I stood there and I just cried. I couldn't stop looking at the casket. Bill had meant so much to me as a friend. For the first time in this business I had met somebody whom I could call at any time to talk about anything, someone who cared about me and someone I really cared about. We laughed and joked so much together. I think that helped me more than anything, his laugh.

Bill had loved his family so much and embraced his son-in-law as the son he never had. He had wanted grandkids in the worst way, but he didn't live to see Eric and Lauren's twin boys, Billy and Miles, born September 1997. After Bill's death, Eric picked up the relationship with us where Bill had left off; he said he knew it was what his father-in-law would have wanted him to do, and Eric's done a marvelous job for us since then and been a true friend.

Still, I miss Bill's laugh. We all miss him.

Back in California, Darryl's mom continued to suffer, but she kept her pain to herself, hiding it in the pages of the journal she wrote in each day. When we read it after her death we understood that she had wanted to shield her children, to protect them from what she was going through. The radiation made her sick, and I think after a while she just decided she'd had enough and it was time to quit treatment. She considered her disease a matter between her and God, who had always kept an eye out for her. Her children were in her prayer thoughts, which she penned daily.

In a way, though, she made it tougher on Darryl and his brothers and sisters by trying to hide her illness, because by the time they found out, she was nearly gone.

At the Yankees' prodding, Darryl and I took the kids and went to Puerto Rico in early November so he could play in the winter league there; apparently team management hadn't seen enough of his game to be convinced during the course of the championship season. We spent Thanksgiving in Puerto Rico, the first away from home for either of us. Darryl stuck it out for a while, and he was killing the ball, hitting something like twelve home runs in thirteen games. So then he told me, "You know what? We're leaving. They've seen me play," and we headed home.

We got back in December, and Darryl's mom was going downhill fast. No one in their family had ever experienced cancer, so none of them knew what to expect. I'd lost my grandmother (my mom's mother) to breast cancer when I was eighteen, so I knew a little of what being around someone dying of cancer was like, but none of them did. What added to her children's devastation was their mother's refusal to opt for medical care. She wanted to be at home, but she wasn't inter-ested in a nurse coming in to look after her. When it got so she couldn't move around anymore, Darryl would carry her back and forth from the bedroom to the bathroom. In the end, when her care was more than we could handle, a hospice nurse would come in and help, but it seemed she lost more ground each day.

We got a hospital bed in and tried to make Mom as comfortable as we could. It was only about an hour's drive from our home to Mom's, and we were in the habit of coming down on Saturday night so we could be close to our church for Sunday morning. Now we started coming down Thursday or Friday. Charisse would drop me off, and I'd spend the day with my sisters, look-ing after our mother.

Then the nurse started coming each day to see Mom, and right away she sat down and told me and my sisters, "Your mom isn't going to live too much longer – maybe a month, maybe two weeks, maybe two days." She'd seen a lot of people die this way, and she told us to start preparing for it. After that, time seemed to run by so fast. They put her on morphine for her pain, and the nurse showed us how to set up the drip. By the end, we had to place the drip in her mouth, her condition was so bad.

Watching her, I felt so completely helpless. The suffering she had to go through in those last stages was painful for me too. I was right there with her, and to see her pain and know there was nothing I could do about it – that really scared me. It had me scared about life, just thinking that this is what it all comes down to, that death is something we're all going to have to face one day.

Mom held on for another two weeks. During that time, all five of us kids had a chance to see her and say good-bye. She must have understood that her illness made us each feel lonely in our own way, because she told us again and again how much she wanted us to stay together, to support each other.

She died on a Sunday morning, with her children right beside her. She looked at each of us, and we told her everything would be fine, we'd be okay. It was like she was staring at us, so she wouldn't forget our faces. She saved her last look for me. I said, "Mom, it's going to be okay. I'll take care of everything." And then she looked at the girls one more time before she let go.

The viewing was the hardest thing to deal with – harder, I think, than the funeral itself. I'd never seen Darryl cry like that before. He broke down. He totally lost it. It hurt to see him like that.

Mom's death had a major effect on me, and burying her was one of the hardest things I've ever had to face. For a while afterward I didn't know if I could go on.

I was so devastated, because in a way she was all I ever had. She represented all that was really important in life. After we buried her, I lay in bed for two weeks. I couldn't bring myself to get up, or even to eat. I just didn't want to go on anymore. But, knowing the type of person my mom was, she would have been saying, "You've got to move on…" That's when I started realizing that I had to regroup, pick myself back up, and move forward. I had to try to be strong for the family, for my sisters and brothers.

It's over three years now since her death, and I still miss her every day. There are days when I miss her more than usual, special days like her birthday or Mother's Day, when families take their moms out to dinner. Instead, we go sit by our mom's grave and place flowers on it, except that usually I can't be there, so my sisters have to go alone. Those days are the most difficult.

But now, through my own battle with cancer, I've gained an appreciation for the things Mom's life taught me that I might otherwise have missed. I think her biggest secret to a fulfilled life lay in her sense of purpose. You see, she knew who she lived for, and those of us around her knew she knew. My mom centered her life on God and spent it trying to serve him. I think that's what gave her such calmness at the end.

I've always looked on my mom as a teacher – not someone who used a lot of words, but someone who got on with things and taught through example. That's how she always was. And without her even knowing it, her dying held a lesson for us children too. It was her final statement on the art of living.

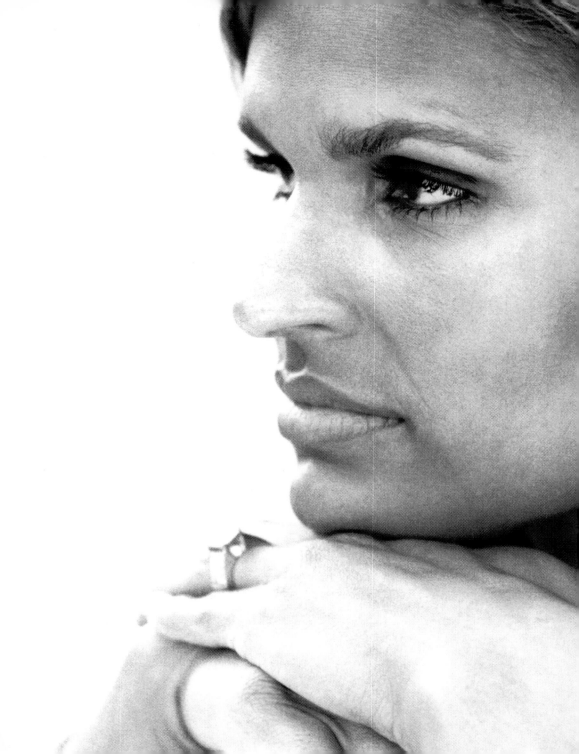

CHAPTER III

CUT OPEN

"I wish I could have broken down and cried,
so he could have told me, 'It's going to be okay.'
But I couldn't, because he was the one
going through it, not me."

"More than anything, I just wanted
to get the whole thing over with."

Friday, October 2, 1998, was Media Day at the Strawberrys. It was the day Darryl and I left for Columbia-Presbyterian Medical Center, the day before his scheduled surgery, and it seemed like every media type east of the Mississippi had made it to our Cedar Street address in Fort Lee to see us off.

Cedar isn't a large street, and satellite trucks and reporters' cars choked our neighbors' driveways and effectively blocked the traffic. Camera crews and journalists stood on the sidewalk,

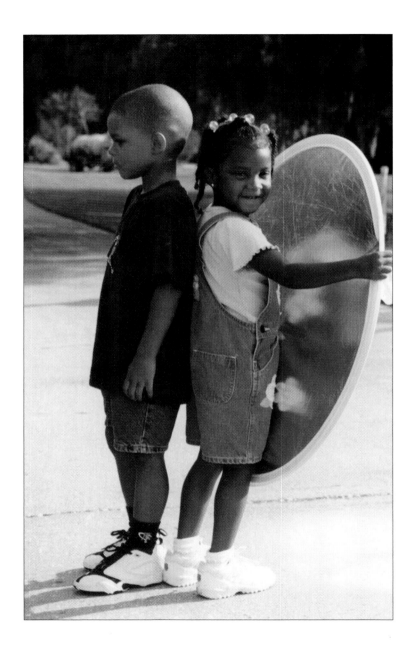

waiting for us to come out. I felt sorry for the people who lived around us and wondered how they would get to work through that circus.

Inside the house, the phone rang nonstop. I had a zillion voice-mail messages. I'd kept our two kids, Jordan, four, and Jade, three, home from their preschool. Thankfully, both of them seemed blissfully unaware of the tension and commotion around them. They knew their daddy was going to the hospital, but they were at peace with the explanation he'd given them: "Daddy's got to get a booboo taken out of his stomach…"

So while Nana and a friend of mine looked after them, I tried to take care of last-minute details and to hold myself together. I did my best to avoid looking out the windows onto the street; whenever I did, I felt a little panicky. I told myself not to be scared, to be strong for Darryl. That was the best way I could see to hold off the whirlwind.

We did two interviews before leaving the house. The first was with ESPN, and after that a crew from NBC came in. They set up a satellite hookup with their reporter Jim Gray, who was with the Yankees in Texas, and with Eric Davis, out in Los Angeles. After Eric and I answered questions and talked back and forth a few minutes, they gave me the opportunity to tape a message for the team. I told the guys that I was with them, even though I wasn't playing. At the end, I pointed into the camera and did my best to glare, but I think I more or less grinned. Then I gave the team my instructions for Game 3 of our Division Series against the Rangers: "Go get 'em tonight. Get 'em!"

Speaking of the team, it touched me deeply to see the way the guys reacted to my condition. When Joe Torre broke the news of my cancer to them in the clubhouse Thursday afternoon, only hours before Game 2, guys cried. Everyone took the news hard, but I think it was especially tough for my good friend and long-time teammate David Cone. Most of the players couldn't seem to believe that I had been in so much pain for so long and hadn't ever said anything about it.

I'd had a chance on Thursday to speak briefly by phone with Torre and Andy Pettitte, who was starting on the mound in Game 2, and had told them I expected the team to take care of business. I also asked Pettitte to pray for me, and he assured me they all would do that. Later that night, on ESPN's "SportsCenter," the team sent me a get-well message. Tim Raines, who would end up splitting designated hitter duties with Chili Davis for the playoffs, spoke for the team, letting me know they were behind me "as a family." I really appreciated that.

But now it was Friday: time to face the music.

I don't really remember what I said once I stepped outside. I think the gist of what I told those reporters was that I wanted people to know I was going to be all right, that this wasn't going to be easy for me, but that I'd come through okay. There'd been rumors flying around about my condition, and I wanted to dispel any myths. I also remember crying in front of the cameras, which isn't something I do very often. I guess I was just dealing with a lot of feelings and emotions and practical things all at the same time, and maybe, like Charisse, I was trying too hard to be brave. I think we both wanted to shield each other.

I know this sounds like a contradiction, but I never doubted the outcome of my surgery. From the time Charisse had broken the news of my diagnosis to me and I'd asked, "What's next?" to the moment I went into the operating room, I felt at peace about my future. It's not something I can explain, but it was definitely there – a deep assurance that my life wasn't in my hands in the first place, and that I would be taken care of.

And, really, the outlook was good. The doctors had sounded positive when they told us my chances for complete recovery, and I knew that my physical fitness gave me an edge going into surgery. So even though both of us were dealing with frayed nerves and strained emotions, as we left for the hospital we wanted to communicate that optimism. We were going to tackle this disease and beat it – neither of us doubted that.

From Darryl's hospital room you could see out across the Hudson River. It was a beautiful view. I had to remind myself that we weren't in a hotel. But that illusion didn't last long, because shortly after we got there, the doctors arrived to talk to us, and then in came the nurses and started sticking needles into Darryl. They drew blood and went about their procedures, with me hovering over them to make sure they didn't screw things up. Even Dr. LaPook, who had cleared his weekend schedule in order to be on hand for Darryl's surgery, commented at one point, "Darryl, does your wife have a medical background?"

Once, I left the room for a moment and when I returned, Darryl had blood streaming down his arm. Apparently a nurse was having a hard time getting the needle to go in where she wanted it…

By the end of the day both Charisse and I were exhausted. We'd been through so much in such a short period – media, doctors, nurses, medication. And that was only the beginning. More than anything, I just wanted to get the whole thing over with. I had to take the Colo-Lyte again that evening so that my colon would be cleaned out by the morning, which is when the surgery was to take place.

They pulled a bed into my room for Charisse, and we both fell asleep. We were just too wiped out to do a lot of talking or anything.

We hugged and said we loved each other. I said, "Everything's going to be okay" – the words we'd repeated to each other so often during those days before the surgery. And then we both lay down and slept.

I wish now that I could have broken down and cried, so he could have told me, "It's going to be okay." I wanted to tell him, "I'm mad! I don't want this to happen!" But I couldn't, because he was the one going through it, not me. So I didn't let myself cry.

I think, though, if our roles had been reversed, he would have let me break down.

Saturday morning started early. My surgery was supposed to begin at seven or eight, so I had to be ready to roll in good time. The nurses came in, did their thing, gave me something to help me relax, and then left. And then we met the "Dream Team" – that's what everyone was calling the surgeons and doctors who were looking after me. There must have been about eleven of them in the room. These guys were the best: the best surgeon, the best anesthesiologist, the best colon and heart guys – they were all there. No question, I got the red-carpet treatment (even if they substituted rubber gloves for kid leather). You couldn't have asked for better care from a group of men who intended to slice you open and cut out sixteen inches of your intestine.

Before they wheeled Darryl to the operating room, we had a few minutes alone, which gave us a chance to pray together. Then I walked beside the gurney as far as they'd let me.

Obviously, I wasn't allowed to be with him during the surgery, and even if I had been, I don't think I would have wanted to see them cut him open. But leaving him, I felt so helpless. I couldn't help thinking, God, what are they going to do to him?

The surgery lasted four hours. There was nothing for me to do but wait. Thankfully, I had company. Two of my girlfriends were there, and Nana came by for a while. And then there was George. Mr. Steinbrenner was there with me during the whole surgery. I knew he cared about Darryl, but that said more to me than any words could.

We sat, chatted, ate lunch, sat some more. Four hours is a long time when there's so much at stake. All I could think was, God, please don't let him have a bag. Please. I was so worried they wouldn't be able to reconnect his colon and would have to do a temporary colostomy, which would then mean more surgery later.

But when the surgeons came out after the operation, they had the best news for me: the surgery had gone extremely well.

No one wanted to sound overly confident, but everyone agreed Darryl's chances for recovery looked great. I could breathe.

At least until I saw Darryl. When they brought him out of surgery and moved him into Intensive Care, he looked terrible – tubes everywhere. I stayed by his side for the afternoon. He was still totally out of it. Being there in Intensive Care was awful; everyone around him seemed to be dying. I saw one guy all bandaged up. I guessed he had gunshot wounds, but when I asked, nobody would say.

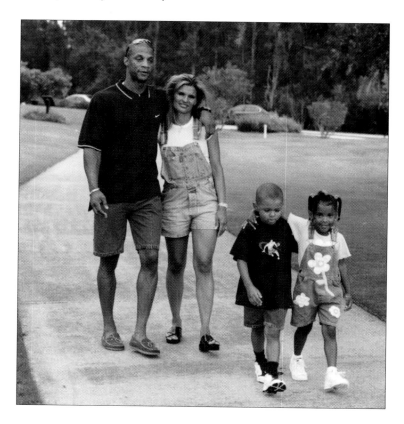

Darryl came to that evening. He wanted me to stay with him for the night, but that wasn't possible. I went home to be with the kids.

Lying there in Intensive Care, I felt groggy and out of it. But I knew one thing: I was a lucky man, with so many things to be thankful for. Sure, this was the last place I ever expected to find myself – I'm an athlete; there's never supposed to be anything wrong with me – and of course I'd been looking forward to post-season play. But I'd been there before, and had two rings to prove it, so it wasn't like I'd never felt the thrill of winning. Somehow the only thing that really seemed to matter was being alive.

In a sense, this wasn't the first time I'd been cut open. How many times before had I been under the knife, my life cut open for all to see and judge? I didn't care to count. Too many times in my life my demons have gotten the better of me, and I've had to face the humiliation of being made a public spectacle. And yet just as often, it seems, I've felt the hand of God pulling me up out of those low places.

And so, lying there in the hospital, the only words that seemed to make sense were "Thank you, God."

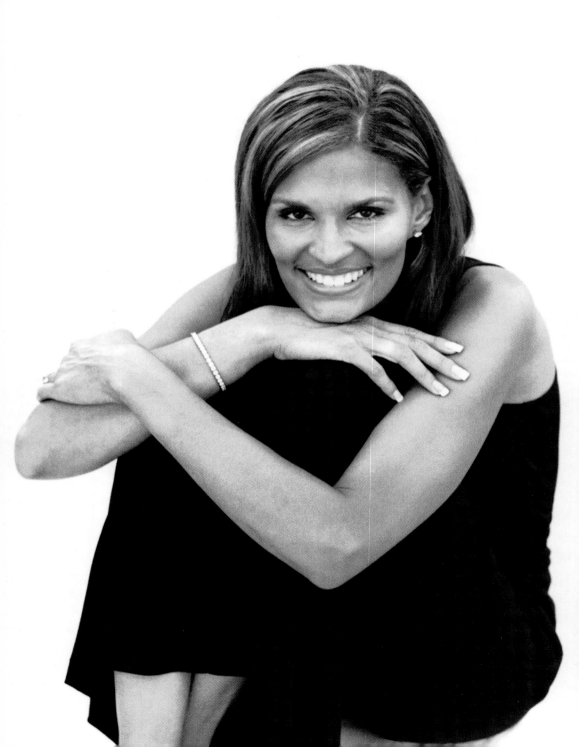

CHAPTER IV

ROMANCE AND
ROLLER COASTERS

"She was definitely different."

"My mom said, 'Call him. It's not like
you're going to marry him, so what's the big deal?
Besides, he has a sparkle in his eyes.'"

H e was wearing a suit. Pale yellow, almost ivory. And some
kind of very colorful shirt. It was the shirt that caught my
eye and made me turn to him the moment I walked into the
room. I couldn't stop myself. I rushed to him and fell into his –
Well, not exactly.

The part about the shirt and suit is true, but the rest of the
story needs a bit of explanation.

Darryl and I first met at a party for Eric Davis's twenty-ninth
birthday, May 29, 1991. All I knew when some friends of mine

asked me to go with them was that we were going to a party at the Beverly Center (in Beverly Hills, where else?) for some baseball player. So I walked in there with my little invitation card, not knowing anyone besides the friends I was with. And not knowing a thing about baseball either; the game had never interested me much.

The party started, and I was on the dance floor with one of the guys. We hadn't been dancing long when someone behind me tapped me on my shoulder. I leaned back to see who it was, and that's when I first took notice of Darryl, a man I'd never seen before in my life. I was still looking over my shoulder, trying to ask what he wanted, when someone else came running up to him. It was obvious that, whoever he was, he was a pretty popular guy.

Actually, I was a bit annoyed at him for interrupting my dance, and I didn't like it much that a minute later he cut in on my partner. I was wearing a hat, which he promptly removed from my head and perched on his own. I thought, Who does this guy think he is? So there I was, about to dance with the man in the pale yellow suit. Maybe he shouldn't have smiled…

She was wearing a black jacket and jeans, I think.

The jacket was red. I wore a black one for our first date.

Well, Charisse is better at details. But I definitely remember the hat. The point is, I thought she looked very attractive. Of all the people at that party, she was the only one I really wanted to talk to. A lot of girls were trying to get with me, but I wasn't interested in giving them much attention. At the time, I wasn't involved with anyone; I was still reeling from my breakup with my first wife, Lisa, and all the publicity around it. Further, I'd only recently begun to face the shallowness of my life and my lack of inner peace, and that had led me to open my heart to God in a way I'd never experienced before. My perspective on life had radically changed, and I was seeing things totally differently.

The last thing I wanted was to get tangled in another dead-end, destructive relationship. But at the same time I was praying for someone different – someone kind, loving, and understanding, whom God would send into my life. Maybe I was lonelier than I cared to realize.

The truth is, if it hadn't been Eric's birthday party, I wouldn't have been out that night. But it was his party, and we were close friends, so I turned up.

And there she was, with her hat.

So he cuts in and starts dancing with me. He asks my name and where I'm from, and then his next question is, "Do you like baseball?" The conversation goes something like this:

"Do you like baseball?"

"No. Why?"

"Because that's what I do. I'm a ball player."

"Oh, really?"

"Yeah."

"Who do you play for?"

"The Dodgers."

"Uh huh."

I don't believe him. Why should I? I'm from California, and I know the Dodgers, sort of. So I ask him his name.

"What's your name?"

"Darryl. Darryl Strawberry."

I've heard that name before. I mean, it's not that hard to re-member a ball player named after a soft fruit.

"Oh, yeah. Okay," I manage. "I know who you are. My brother loves you."

"Oh, yeah? Okay."

We dance a while, and then he wants to know, do I cook — and if he came to my apartment in Fullerton, would I make him dinner? I think, I don't cook. That's what I tell him. He tries again. If he drove down to Orange County, would I take him out to dinner? I roll my eyes. "No. I don't think so." Then I add, "But you can come out and take me to dinner."

"Oh, okay," he says.

And then the song is over. I say, "Thanks for the dance," and walk away.

After the party, I waited at the door for Charisse to leave the club. From our brief dance, I knew I wanted to spend more time with her, though I didn't really know why. I guess most of my life I'd been around women with wild, crazy streaks, who liked to hang out and party. Charisse obviously wasn't that type. She was def-initely different. There was something almost naïve about her, a lack of self-awareness, and that drew me to her. Also, I liked her attitude. She wasn't falling all over me – and that was genuinely refreshing.

I wanted her phone number. I'd asked her for it on the dance floor, but she'd hedged and told me she'd give it to me later. So when she came out, I went up to her and asked her for it. She seemed just the slightest bit flustered to see me again. I thought to myself, again, This one is definitely different...

Of course some people had taken note of my dance with Darryl. As I found out later, there were a handful of women in the club who really wanted to be with him. So I had to contend with a bit of jealous whispering going on, but it didn't really faze me since I had no intentions of getting involved with anything – or anybody.

Which is why I wasn't thrilled to see Darryl waiting for me at the door. Our second conversation of the night:

I say, to myself, "Oh, gosh. Him again."

He says, to me, "May I have your number?"

At this, all his little friends swarm around me, munchkin-like, "Oh, give him your number! Give him your number!" (Lollipop Guild members in good standing, all of them.)

"Well, are you going to or not?" Darryl asks.

"No, I've got a better idea – you give me yours."

"Just give me your digits. Please."

"Actually, why don't you just autograph my invitation card, for my brother."

In the end, I gave him a number – but not mine. It was one of my girlfriends'. Then he gave me his, and we said goodnight.

I seriously thought that would be the end of it. But the next morning my girlfriend, whom I'd tipped off about the number thing, rang to say Darryl had called for me. "Oh, well," I said, and left it at that.

A couple months before Eric's party, I had broken up with a boyfriend, and I guess I was a little nervous. I couldn't deny that I felt attracted to Darryl, but I sort of held myself back. Then my friends wanted an explanation why I'd given him someone else's number, and I couldn't come up with a reasonable answer.

I don't know how many times Darryl called my girlfriend that week, but finally I decided I better call him back. This wasn't something I cared to lose a girlfriend over. My mom, who knew of Darryl from seeing him on TV, gave me the final encouragement I needed to pick up the phone: "Call him," she said. "It's not like you're going to marry him, so what's the big deal? Besides, he has a sparkle in his eyes."

I called.

It's about time, was my first thought when I picked up the phone to hear Charisse's voice. Her holding out set a new record, at least in my books. We chatted, and ended up arranging a date for that Sunday night. I agreed to drive from my home in Sherman Oaks out to Fullerton. We planned dinner at Hoff's Bar & Grill.

I hung up with an unusual feeling of anticipation. Something told me Sunday evening was going to be – well, different.

He arrived late. But at least he'd called from his car phone to let me know he was coming. He pulled into the parking lot outside the apartment complex in his red two-seater Mercedes. From the window of my second-floor apartment, I watched him get out. He was wearing a jeans outfit. He came up, knocked on my door, and escorted me to the car.

By the time we got to Hoff's it was already ten o'clock. Closing time. But the owner recognized Darryl and let us in. I ordered a bacon cheeseburger and we had a really nice time there, just the two of us. The whole evening was surprisingly romantic, what with his taking my coat and opening the car door for me and all. (He doesn't do that anymore, but he did then...)

The thing I loved most about our first date was Charisse's lack of pretense. She sat across the table from me, and our conversation flowed so naturally. There was no trace of the charade I'd grown accustomed to over the course of my career, the fake way many people behave around so-called celebrities. I was Darryl, and she was Charisse. And that was beautiful.

He took me back to my apartment and we talked a while longer – family stuff mostly, I think. He told me the team was heading out on a road trip the next day and wanted to know if he could call me while he was away. I told him that would be fine. He gave me a kiss on the cheek, and then left.

My apartment had a balcony at the back, and Darryl's car was parked under it. When I said goodnight to him and closed the door, I had to run across the living room and fight with the blinds so I could see out over the balcony and into the parking lot. I wanted to say good-bye and see him one more time, though I was sure he'd already be gone. But he was there, and as he got into his car, he turned and looked up, and I waved.

Later, discussing that moment, we realized both of us had felt something like a spiritual connection pass between us then. I knew, as I turned away from the window, that I was going to miss Darryl while he was out of town. And he told me over the phone how good it made him feel to see me wave. He called me from his car on the way home to say how much he'd enjoyed the evening.

That road trip, I called Charisse every night. AT&T should have awarded me Preferred Customer status or something by the end of that week – she and I would go on and on for five, six, seven hours at a stretch, talking into the early morning. Obviously, we had a lot to say to each other.

Right from the start, I wanted to be up front about my life and the things I'd been through. Charisse deserved honesty, I knew – and on top of that, her b.s. detector was in great working order. Besides, there weren't many secrets I could reveal to her that weren't already public knowledge. My five-year marriage to Lisa Andrews had been rocky at best; at worst it had been a nightmare. From 1987 on, we went through periods of legal separation, but it wasn't until January 1990, when I was arrested for sticking a handgun in her face during an all-out fight, that our relationship reached the point of complete meltdown. We had wounded each other too many times, physically and emotionally.

My marriage was in ruins, and this time neither of us I had the strength, or the inclination, to try to piece it back together. Our divorce wasn't finalized until October 1993, but our marriage ended long before.

There were other things too: My career with the Mets, the team I'd made my major league debut with, ended on an off note with me checking into New York's Smithers Institute for alcohol rehabilitation. So by the time the Dodgers signed me as a free agent on November 8, 1990, my checkered past was common knowledge.

This was the man Charisse was getting involved with, and I wanted to be fair to her; if there were things that needed an explanation, I wanted to be the one doing the explaining. But at the same time, I didn't want to burden her unnecessarily with the wrongs of my past. Although the change was only recent, I had started on a new path – away from the lifestyle and influences that had scarred me so badly and toward a relationship with God that would, I hoped, lay the groundwork for a new foundation for my life.

Ironically, it was my first wife's uncle, Bill Payne, who had talked me into spending a few days at the Morris Cerullo Convention Center in Anaheim only days after Lisa and I had gone through our big fight. Morris Cerullo was known for his preaching, and for the way he could reach people whose spirits were worn ragged. I went, and experienced for the first time an inkling of what God's love could be like. Finally it began to dawn on me how far gone I was and how radically my life needed an overhaul.

As the 1991 season got underway, I adjusted to playing in a new town with new teammates and new fans, but my biggest adjustment of all had to do with learning to play with the new person I was becoming. The peace growing inside me almost scared me sometimes, I was so unaccustomed to it. But it also gave me the assurance that my life could be different, that even though my problems wouldn't just pack up and go away, I now had Someone far more powerful than myself – or my problems – to help fight my battles.

Those phone calls during Darryl's road trip were more important for our future than I think either of us realized. As we talked about our pasts and our dreams for the future, I felt more and more certain that meeting Darryl hadn't just been a chance thing. There was a depth to our conversations that I'd never known before with anyone else. I knew he'd had a turbulent marriage, but he was straightforward when talking about Lisa, and the love he felt for their two children showed in his voice when he told me about them. And he listened, genuinely interested, when I talked about my background.

I was born January 21, 1967, in Salt Lake City, Utah, to Walter and Aleta Simon. My parents were both nineteen when they married. Mom was twenty when she had me. We're a biracial family; Mom is white, and Dad is black. Dad, who grew up in California, was playing basketball for the University of Utah. When I was about two years old, he finished school and was drafted by the Seattle Supersonics, and we moved out to Orange County, California, not far from where Nana lived.

At that time Orange County was predominantly white, so during my grade school years most of my friends were white simply because there were very few black kids around. Once in a while some kid would see me with my mom and ask me if I was adopted, which I always thought was strange since I look a lot like her, only darker of course.

Really, though, I can't say I ever gave much thought to how I "fit in," in terms of my color. My parents taught me to be confident and have self-esteem. They always told me, "You are who you are. You have the best of both worlds." When I was older they stressed, "Don't get caught up in race. Date whom you want to date – it doesn't matter if he's Mexican, white, black, Chinese, or whatever." They were adamant about combating racism. All the same, perhaps because of my father, I identified best with black men and sort of always assumed I'd wind up marrying one.

After starting his professional career in Seattle, Dad moved on to play for the Los Angeles Stars in the ABA. When I was about eight years old, he signed with a team in Sweden, so we moved to Europe and lived there for a year while Dad finished his career. And that's where my brother Miles was born. I was so happy to have a sibling and was all over him right away, making his bottle, changing his diapers, fixing his hair. I couldn't wait for him to grow up so we could play together.

Going to school in Sweden presented me with challenges. I caught on to the language quite quickly (though I've since forgotten it all), but there were some things I just couldn't adjust to – like when we went on fieldtrips in the summer and everyone would swim naked. I'd tell my mom, "Don't make me go to school today. I can't go!"

We returned to California after that year. For the most part I had a happy childhood, getting involved in lots of extracurricular activities at school – softball, basketball, volleyball, going to "charm school" and getting into modeling, that kind of thing. Life wasn't perfect, though. My parents had their share of fights, and things weren't always smooth in our home.

One thing I can say is that both my parents took a lot of interest in my upbringing and did their best to teach me responsibility. My dad, in particular, was very structured and always insisted that I do my homework and chores every night. Even when I was in high school, fifteen or sixteen years old, I can still remember him waking me up from a deep sleep at three o'clock in the morning to load the dishwasher, because I hadn't bothered to do it before I went to bed. He'd especially waited until I was sound asleep before he got me out of bed. It was his way of getting a point across.

My parents stayed together until I was fifteen. After their divorce, I ended up staying with my dad and Nana, who'd always been close to my mom. So actually Dad and Mom stayed on good terms, out of their love for Miles and me.

Right from my earliest years Nana had played a big role in my life, and she was very special to me. She'd moved in with us back when I was in eighth grade, so I was used to having her around all the time. But after Dad and Mom split up, Nana really became a second mother to me. She was right by my side as I grew into a young woman. When it comes to personalities, Nana and my father are a lot alike, and I know they're the source of my strong will and self-confidence.

Dad continued to set standards for me. He'd made me wait until high school before allowing me to wear makeup, and I knew dating was out of the question until I turned sixteen. When I did start going out in the evenings, he'd be up waiting for me when I got home. If I was late, I could always expect consequences. One time I had a volleyball tournament at a crosstown school the next day, and he dropped me off there but made me take the bus home as a punishment.

Through high school, I enjoyed playing basketball and volleyball, which I played well enough to get into Cal State Fullerton on a scholarship. So I played volleyball while majoring in communications. I had visions of becoming a sportscaster, following in the footsteps of my idol, Jane Kennedy. My dad, though, always thought I'd make a good lawyer, and he encouraged me to switch my focus to studying criminal justice. He was working in administration as a supervisor at Juvenile Hall. So I changed majors and got a job as a deputy probation counselor, working with juvenile delinquents – a far cry from my previous work in retail and occasional modeling jobs. That's the stage I was at when I first met Darryl, but it wouldn't take me long to figure out I didn't like my new job, or to make the switch back to my communications major.

When Darryl got back into town after that road trip, we started spending serious time together. I'll never forget the first Dodgers game I attended. My dad and Miles went with me, along with one of my girlfriends. Darryl had left us tickets for seats in the players' family section. That was my introduction to LA, the city where everyone's watching – all the time. After the game I was supposed to meet Darryl, and while I was waiting for him, I could feel an awful lot of eyes on me. He took me to the players' lot, a fenced-in area where they all parked. A crowd of kids pressed against the fence, trying to catch a glimpse of their heroes, and Darryl walked over to the gate and signed autographs. I didn't know it then, but that was something Darryl did after every home game. It was something that impressed me about him – not that I needed impressing, but there was something reassuring in seeing small things like that, which spoke volumes for his character and heart.

In July, he took me to the Six Flags Magic Mountain theme park, and we enjoyed a great time together, going on all the crazy rides. I realized that day for the first time just how big a star Darryl was: we were followed everywhere; it seemed everyone wanted to be around Darryl.

He did his best to ease my transition into the spotlight I'd have to share with him if we stayed together. "Don't let this bother you. Don't get caught up in that. Just ignore that woman over there who's calling my name; don't let it get to you." He was always looking out for me and helping me adjust.

When Darryl said he wanted to introduce me to his children, Darryl Jr. and Diamond Nicole, I wasn't sure how I'd respond to them. Here I was, falling in love with their father, and I thought, Oh God, he has these two kids with somebody else whom he loved at one time… But the kids turned out to be great. DJ was six and Diamond was three at the time, and both of them were so cute. We took them to the batting cages and the mini-golf course at the Camelot arcade, and then stopped for ice cream at Baskin-Robbins before heading back to his place.

Once Darryl brought the kids into my life, I tried to be a friend to them. I knew I would never be able to take their mom's place, and that wasn't something I wanted to do. We lived only fifteen minutes from Lisa's house, and the children spent a good deal of time with us. We'd go shopping together, and I'd take them to the movies or watch TV with them. They sat with me at Dodgers games, and when we could, they'd come with us on road trips. I couldn't help feeling grateful for the way they accepted me.

In September 1992 Darryl underwent surgery to fix a ruptured disc in his spine. He moved from his home in Encino to his mom's house for his recovery. We'd been dating for over a year by then and our conversations about marriage grew more and more serious. So that December we decided to move in together, at least for the next baseball season. We found a house in Glendale and got settled in.

We fell in love, married, and started a family, and it's been "happily ever after." That's what I'd like to be able to say, but that's not what happened.

Back when I first met Charisse, I was going through a very difficult and stressful time in my life. Even though I'd decided to turn my life over to God, I wanted an easy release from my problems. It didn't take long for me to pick up a bottle. Before I knew it, my alcoholism was back in force, and once I started drinking again, drugs seemed like the logical next step. Soon I was right back doing the same things that had brought about my downfall in New York – only this was worse. With the Mets, I'd been known to take amphetamines ("uppers") to compensate for my almost permanent hangover, and I'd "messed around" with cocaine, too. In Los Angeles, though, my cocaine abuse eclipsed any past drug-related problems. Like every drinker and user on the face of the earth, I gave in to my addictions in an attempt to escape the demons lurking inside of me.

Of course, having come out and declared my newfound faith in God, I had left myself wide open for ridicule. I mean, once God comes into a person's life, then that person's problems are solved, right? Wrong! Nowhere have I ever read that that's supposed to be the case. When you decide for God, there are no guarantees. It's sad, but many people don't understand that, and they're quick to judge someone who backslides: "Well, I thought God was supposed to be fighting your battles. What's going on?" In a way, reactions like that are perfectly understandable, but I've come to understand that following God really has nothing to do with me being perfect, and everything to do with the attitude of my heart. I don't want to live a bad life; I want the fruits of my life to be good ones. My intent needs to be always focused on doing right, on choosing the right road. And I have to believe that when I fall – and I will fall; *that's* guaranteed – God won't desert me if I work to set right the wrong I've done.

Sometimes it's hard for me to believe that, but luckily there's someone right beside me who believes for me when I'm unsure. Her name is Charisse. Even though she didn't talk a lot about it, I know it was her strong faith that helped her through the storms brought on by my bouts of drinking and using.

From the beginning of our relationship, it was clear to both Charisse and me that something very special was taking place between us. Within half a year, we knew it without a doubt: we belonged together. It was obvious that, at some point, we were going to get married. We had a lot of fun talking over our plans for our future, which helped me get through the disappointment of missing all but thirty-two games of the 1993 baseball season on account of my back injury.

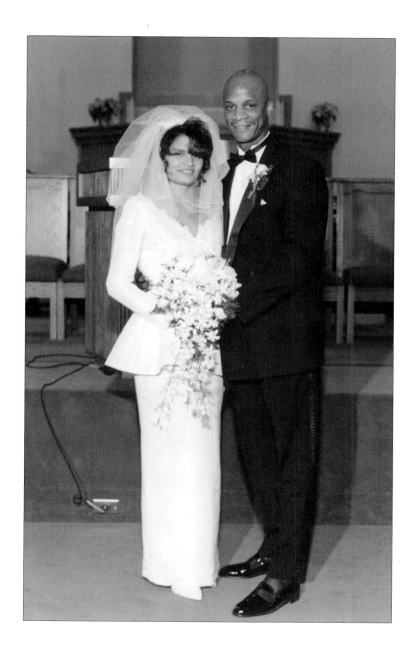

Darryl proposed and gave me a ring on Thanksgiving Day 1993. We set a wedding date for November 12, 1994, and I got started putting lists together. To add to my excitement, I was expecting our first child, due in March 1994. It was a happy time for both of us. Then, a couple weeks after our engagement, Darryl came home one evening and said, "Charisse, this isn't right. We're not living right. We've got to get married. Now." I looked at him. "Now?" I had especially wanted us to wait until after the baby arrived, so that I could fit into my beautiful, fitted wedding dress, but Darryl insisted we needed to marry as soon as possible. So we shifted gears.

I called Nana and my godmother, Margery Leonard (ever since my childhood, she and her husband, Paul, my godfather – "Ma" and "Pa," I call them – have been a special part of my life, and Darryl and I had asked them to be our baby's godparents as well), and I told them, "I have a week to plan my wedding. Darryl and I are getting married December 3rd." And that was it. With their help, everything came together. The mother of one of my good friends is a seamstress, and she made my dress in just five days. We cut the guest list from three hundred to thirty and were married at my home church in Orange County, Friendship Baptist, by the pastor of St. Stephen Baptist, where Darryl and I are members. Darryl had told me he wasn't going to wear a tux, which disappointed me. But he was only kidding, so it turned out okay. The wedding was followed by a reception at the Ritz Carlton in Laguna Niguel, where we then spent our one-night "honeymoon."

We married on a Friday, spent the next day with family, and then went to church on Sunday. Neither of us has looked back since. And in my heart I know we never will.

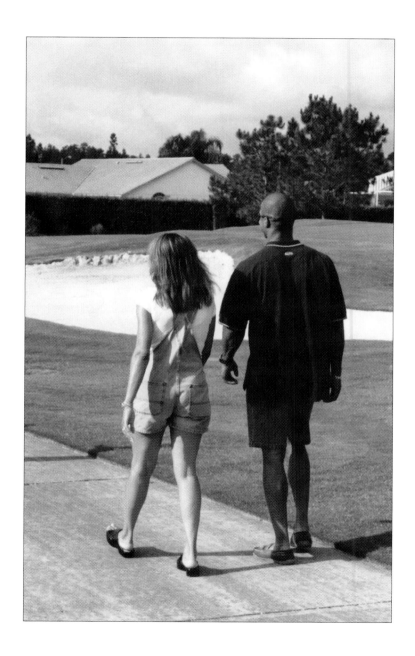

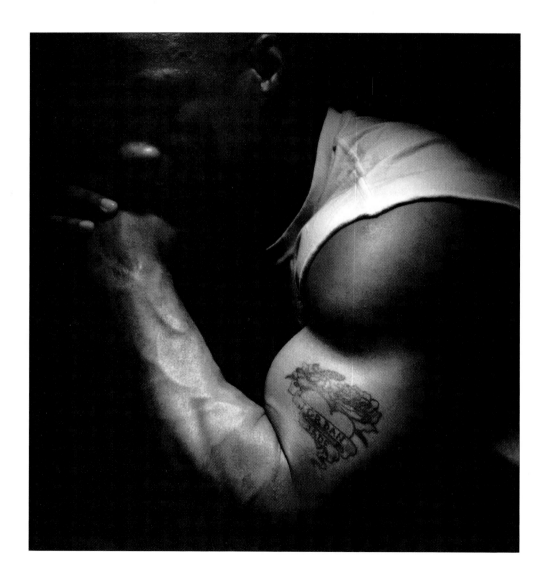

CHAPTER V

BREAKING THE CYCLE

"It hurts me to see him
misunderstood, or misinterpreted."

"It's a force, an evil force, that tries to
get you in a death grip, and it takes an
awful lot of strength to break out of it."

When the news of Darryl's cancer hit the media, we were bowled over by the huge wave of sympathy and support. Hundreds of people wrote to tell us they understood what we were going through, to share stories from their own families about facing cancer.

There's no question that we felt uplifted by the prayers and thoughts of so many, and I would wish the same experience for anyone having to deal with a situation like that. But there's another side to this as well. I don't know if I'll be able to explain it the way I'd like to, but I'm going to try; I think it's very important that I do.

Cancer, like all potentially fatal diseases, is a killer without conscience. It doesn't care if you're rich or and poor, white or black, young or old. Once it strikes, you're at its mercy, and your only hope lies in uncovering it before it takes complete hold. People know this. They understand. And so when someone is discovered to have cancer, they naturally rally and offer whatever support they can, even if that only means voicing sympathy.

I know another disease that's a lot like cancer. It's called alcoholism, and in some way it affects virtually every family in this country. People know this, but they don't understand. Or maybe they just don't want to. When someone comes out and admits to having an addiction, most turn away, pretend they didn't hear. Some get upset and use it as an occasion to throw stones.

In our family, I've seen cancer – I lost a grandmother and my mother-in-law to it, and I came close to losing Darryl – and I've seen alcoholism, too. I know how similar these two diseases are. I know that no one who is treated for cancer is ever completely "safe" from it again; I know that no one who has ever been dependent on alcohol can ever be completely "safe" again, either. But it doesn't do me any good knowing these things unless other people know them too.

It's tempting to think of alcoholism as a "mistake" resulting from a series of bad choices, or from a lack of good role models. I once thought that way. Now that I've learned to think of it as a disease – one that research has shown gets passed down from generation to generation in the genes of at-risk families – I'm more aware of what it takes to beat the odds. Recovering alcoholics don't need sympathy or greeting cards, they need a determined personal attitude. But they also need support from people who understand their sickness and work with them to master it. People who will stand by them, no matter what happens, so that even when they relapse, someone is there to stop their fall and help them start over.

"Well, yeah, we all make mistakes, but how many chances does a person get?" Many people, it seems, like to throw around those kind of lines. They act as if we each have a "screw-up quota," and once we've hit our limit, well, that's just too bad. Chalk up another strikeout.

To say that someone doesn't deserve another chance at redemption – that stumps me. History is loaded with examples of people who screwed up big time, but who nonetheless got another shot at starting over. Sunday school heroes like Moses and King David, who played huge roles in the history of their people, showed that they too had feet of clay: Moses started his career as a leader by committing murder; King David had a crush on the wife of his chief army captain and, in order to get in bed with her, engineered a battle so that his captain ended up killed in action…

Jesus of Nazareth, one of the best storytellers of all time, told a story to show that people are not always as "righteous" as they might like to think. It goes something like this: Two men go into the temple to pray. One is a Pharisee, a big-name religious leader, and the other a tax collector, a man everyone loves to hate. The Pharisee starts to pray, thanking God that he isn't a waste of space or an adulterer like so many other people.

"I fast twice a week and give away ten percent of everything I get," he goes on. He winds up by saying how grateful he is that he isn't a loser like the tax collector standing in the back of the temple. Then the tax collector says his prayer. He doesn't even take his eyes off the floor as he pleads, "God, have mercy on me. I'm a sinner."

After telling this story, Jesus pointed out that it was the tax collector, not the self-righteous Pharisee, who went home feeling at peace with his God…

Whenever Darryl talks about his problems with alcohol and drug abuse, my protective instincts show up. It hurts me to see him misunderstood, or misinterpreted, but at the same time I know that when he speaks about his battles it encourages many who share similar struggles. They understand that fighting an addiction is like fighting a war: chances are, you won't win every battle, but that doesn't mean you lie down and surrender.

Through good days and bad, Darryl and I continue to grow in our understanding of what Jesus meant when someone asked him if seven times should be the limit of forgiveness, and he answered, "No. Seventy times seven." And both of us know that in the end what matters most is not what other people think of us, but where we stand in the eyes of God.

Some things you just don't forget. And some things you can't forget — even if you'd rather not have to remember them. The night my dad left us is one of those things. I was still in junior high, not much over thirteen, but I think a part of my childhood ended that night.

Dad had been out drinking, as usual, and returned late. He came into the house and start arguing with Mom about something, and their shouts woke us all up. It's hard to explain exactly what happened after that, but somehow as a family we knew we couldn't take it anymore. We'd seen enough, put up with enough.

My father (his name is Henry) was a postal worker, but we might as well have been on welfare. He was an addicted gambler and a drinker. That pretty much took care of his paycheck — and, when he had his way, most of Mom's as well. When he was home, which wasn't very often, we tried to stay clear of him. He would come to the house and crash, and we wouldn't see him until late in the afternoon, which was when he got up to go to work.

I don't remember ever talking to my father about the things fathers and sons supposedly communicate about. There was no relationship between him and his boys, no love. When my brother Ronnie got in trouble with the police and had to appear in Juvenile Court, the judge asked my father what he should do with his son, and my dad told him: "I don't want him back. You can keep him, for all I care." Mom came down later and brought Ronnie home.

It seemed like the only times Dad paid us any attention was when he was kicking us around — and he seemed to find a reason for that on a regular basis. He'd beat me for the least little offense, make me take my shirt off and whip me with an extension cord. But worse than that was having to listen to him go after my mother, who did her best to hold her marriage together for the sake of us children.

I guess it was only a matter of time before everything crashed and burned.

Michael was already in the kitchen with Mom, who had Dad screaming in her face, by the time Ronnie and I got out of bed. Michael, in tenth grade and the oldest of us, did the talking. I remember my knees knocking together as I listened to him. "Why don't you just get your stuff, get out of here, and leave us alone?" How could he dare stand up to my father like that? Then Dad exploded and started in on him. He was talking completely crazy, saying he was going to kill us all, but we weren't buying it. Ronnie and I went to grabbing things – a frying pan, a kitchen knife, a baseball bat – and we told our father we were with Michael: nothing was going to happen to Mom, or to Michael, or to any of us.

I don't think Dad ever expected to be challenged, because in the end he backed down. He left the house that night, and not long afterward Mom got a divorce. Our family life, for what it was worth, was over…

There's nothing very original about that story; it's one that gets repeated every day in homes all across America. But just because the plot is a common one doesn't mean the pain of that kind of breakup is any less.

Every boy wants and needs a dad – not just someone who played a role in your being born, but someone who cares and loves you, and spends time with you. It's true that before my dad left us, he used to take us to the park sometimes, and we brothers would watch him play ball. He had a reputation throughout the city for being a hard-throwing, hard-hitting quarterback, and a tough-to-hit baseball pitcher who swung a wicked bat. In the sports department, Dad was "the man." But those are some of the only nice memories I have of him; the rest are associated with hurt – and fear.

I knew the effects of Dad's addictions firsthand, and I knew the pain and grief he caused my mother. So from the time I was old enough to realize that something wasn't quite right about my father – from the time it registered that there were people with fathers who didn't beat them over freak things – I swore to myself that, if I ever had kids, I would raise them differently. There was no way I was ever going to be an abusive drunk. I had no idea then just how high the odds stacked against me really were.

In high school, sports became a real outlet for me. I lettered in football, basketball, and baseball. That meant I had little time for much else, even for girlfriends, let alone getting caught up in some of the wilder things going on around school. I smoked a bit of pot and enjoyed my beer when I could get it, but I wasn't much of a party kid; most of the time I was just too tired from playing and training.

It really wasn't until I made it to the Mets that I took my first serious steps on the road toward alcoholism. In the majors, drinking became my way to take the edge off of stress. As long as there was alcohol in my bloodstream, I was relieved of the incredible pressure I felt on my shoulders, the pressure of being someone else's rising star. More important, it was a way to make me feel less alone. Somehow drinking made my problems shrink, at least for a while, and the familiar ache of loneliness grew smaller in proportion to my level of intoxication. I would drink with the guys on the team, but I would also drink in my hotel room, by myself, just to have the feeling of alcohol in my system.

Later, when I married Lisa, my drinking bouts spilled into our life and played a big part in tearing our relationship to pieces. I didn't know it then, but I was following a script handed down from generation to generation in my family. My father's father was an alcoholic who, according to some family members, beat his wife to death (no charges were ever pressed). My dad grew up without either parent around; he was raised by his grandmother. He must have been tremendously affected by this, because he picked up where his father left off and kept the cycle of abuse going after he started his own family. When he left us, the stage was set for us boys to follow his lead. Much as I swore I was going to be different, when it came my turn I stepped right into line — and the cycle got set for another round.

It took me a long time to learn that alcoholism is a disease and to treat it like one. It's as much of a disease as cancer, only in some ways it's even more deadly. Like cancer, it grows in you, unnoticed at first, but eventually it will take over your whole body unless you do something to stop it. But unlike cancer, which attacks your physical self, alcoholism goes after your soul as well. It's a force, an evil force, that tries to get you in a death grip, and it takes an awful lot of strength to break out of it. Actually, you never do. The most you can learn is that by yourself you are completely helpless, and that it's only through the help of a Higher Power – and a set of strong friends – that you stand any chance at all.

When I first went public with my drinking problem back in February 1990, I checked into Smithers because I wanted to get back onto the diamond and on with my career. I was sick of the way my drinking was pulling my life apart. It had wrecked my reputation and career with the Mets, and worse, it had torn my marriage right down the middle. But I didn't really have any idea of the amount of resolve and commitment it would take if I intended to stay clean once I'd made it through my twenty-eight days in detox.

I walked out of Smithers – and right back into my broken-down life. My relationship with Lisa was a complete mess, and I felt hopeless about ever getting it back to rights. Too many problems, too many things I didn't have the courage to face. It didn't take long before I sneaked that "first drink," and from there it was a matter of course that my drinking habit kicked in right where I'd left off.

Again, there's nothing out of the ordinary about what I'm saying here. Walk into any Alcoholics Anonymous meeting any-where in the country, and you'll hear the same story repeated over and over. The names and faces change, but the disease stays the same…

When I met Charisse, I was on a path to a new life. I'd turned my life over to God, and for the first time I was learning how to steer myself clear of the pitfalls that I'd stumbled into so many times in my past. It was like I was on a spiritual high, going to church, studying my Bible, and making new friends who could influence my life in a positive way. But despite the peace I was feeling, there were still many hard issues regarding my personal life that I wasn't facing. In a way, I guess you could say I lacked realism. Or maybe it was just that some things were more convenient to hide from than to deal with.

There was a lot of anger pent up inside me, much of which was directed against my dad – or lack of one. I tried hard to ignore it, pretending that it would just go away by itself. Of course, that didn't happen.

My back injury had kept me off the field for the better part of the summer of 1992, and it virtually took away my '93 season. No athlete wants to be sidelined, and I felt particularly frustrated since I'd desperately wanted to rebuild my career in LA. With time on my hands, sitting around waiting for my body to heal, it wasn't long before my demons started their usual whisperings. This time, when I began drinking again, I threw drugs into the mix and started using cocaine seriously for the first time.

Charisse stayed by my side through this. She herself never touched a drink. I, on the other hand, wanted to go out and drink and hang out all the time. She stuck with me and never gave up praying for me. She cared so deeply about me – even I could see that. So when we found out we were going to be parents, our decision to marry came naturally.

Then in March 1994, only a couple months into our marriage, we took our first big hit when the IRS came calling. The accusation: failure to file tax returns for income I'd received between 1986 and 1990 from autograph and memorabilia shows, to the tune of $300,000.

The investigation came as a complete surprise. I had no idea that anything illegal had been going on. After all, card shows were nothing new; people all around baseball – including Hall of Famers – were doing them. A promoter lines up a show, you go sign autographs for a few hours, for which you get a check for ten- or twelve-thousand dollars. Back at the time I'd been involved, I'd had a team of people handling all my financial matters for me, so I had simply assumed that my tax filings were being taken care of professionally and that nothing underhanded was going on. I didn't know then that it was common for people not to report earnings from these types of shows.

When the IRS officials caught wind of the scam, they decided they needed to make an example of someone, and that someone turned out to be me. Knowing I could be facing prison time if I was convicted devastated me. (The way it worked out, in February 1995 I pled guilty to a felony charge and was sentenced at the end of April to six months of home confinement, 100 hours of community service, and a $350,000 fine for tax evasion – nothing I'd ever want to go through again, but it sure beat serving time.) And when you're an alcoholic and a user and all of a sudden your world starts to slide dangerously, there's only one way to handle your problem: start drinking and using. Again.

In my mind, I thought I was being "responsible" with my addictions. After all, they weren't stopping me from doing my job. But it got to the point where I realized I couldn't keep going this way: I was a tired man, tired of trying to outrun my demons, tired of my foul moods, hangovers, and headaches. I kept telling myself, "I'm going to quit." But I just couldn't. I would go clean for a day or two, but then fall right back to drinking and using. In my heart I knew I was a better person than the one I had become, but at the same time I just couldn't figure out why I couldn't control my cravings.

Slowly I began to see how sick I actually was. Once I accepted that, I was able to level with the team and admit what people already knew. My decision to seek help came from deep within me. Charisse had given birth to our son Jordan only four weeks earlier, and I knew I was doing this as much for him and her as for me. But I was scared. I didn't know if I'd ever be able to make headway against my problems, but I knew I had no choice except to try – or die. And that's more or less how I landed up in the Betty Ford Clinic, in Palm Springs, going through treatment for the second time.

Of course, when we made the announcement to the media that I was checking in at Betty Ford, it made headlines. But that couldn't stop me from feeling that a weight was beginning to slip off my shoulders, even though I knew my days as a Dodger were finished.

The next twenty-eight days were filled with learning once again that life could be different from what it had become. There were group sessions and one-on-one counseling. As I went to meetings and heard other addicts share their stories, new hope slowly entered me. Maybe things could really change. In the past, I'd used my addictions as what I thought was the easy way out whenever my problems seemed too tough to deal with. They were a way to escape. My counselors helped me to see that only by confronting the difficult issues in my life would I be able to get clean. They got me writing about the problems that hurt most, the things I'd tried to cover over.

I'm not the kind of guy who goes looking for people to blame for my problems, but one thing my stay at Betty Ford brought out was the feeling of rejection I'd been battling ever since my father quit on us, back when I was a kid. I'd grown up with fantasies, I guess you could call them, of what it would be like to have a dad I could count on for guidance, and who'd spend time teaching me the little things – how to shave, how to judge a high fly ball – too. But those dreams had been replaced with the reality that learning things on your own is often very painful.

There had been times over the years when I'd tried to talk to my dad, but somehow I'd never been able to express to him my part of the pain he'd caused his family. Now, here in the Betty Ford Clinic, part of my rehab was to invite family members to a special session during "family week." I knew there were things I needed to tell my father, and that I had to say them to his face.

Both my brothers came: Michael, who'd served as a police officer but had been forced to retire after taking a bullet during the LA riots, and Ronnie, who knew from his own experiences the hell of my sickness. Charisse was there, too. And then there was Dad. All of us were sitting there, and each of us had issues we were dealing with, but we all shared a piece of the same pain. It's amazing how much pain can be concentrated within a family...

I sat there and told my dad all the things I'd bottled up for years, and he heard me out. He said he was sorry for the things he'd done to hurt us, but that he was a different man now from the one he was then. Things hadn't turned out the way he'd wanted them to, he told me. Listening to him, it suddenly occurred to me that I actually understood my father better than I ever thought I could. The words coming from his mouth sounded so familiar, like so many words I myself had used to try to make sense of my own actions. I understood how he was feeling.

That day, emotionally draining as it was, stands as a kind of milestone along my road to recovery. Once I could express to my father and members of my family the pain I was trying to come to terms with, and also tell them how sorry I was for what my problems put them through, I was able to find forgiveness in my heart.

I don't think the hurt my father caused will ever fade completely, but at least my resentment toward him has evaporated. Even though he never taught me any better, I can't blame him for the poor choices I've made. I can only work to break the cycle, so that my children can be free from its curse. And I have to remember that if I want to receive forgiveness myself, then I have to be the first to forgive – not just once or twice, but over and over again – "seventy times seven." It's what's expected of me, and it's the only way I stand a chance of overcoming the demons of addiction.

In February 1996, my dad was there when we buried Mom. He stood off to one side, not quite sure how he belonged there, watching as the woman he must once have loved was laid to rest. I saw my father at that moment, and all I could feel was pity.

That's a nice way to wrap up talking about a rough time in my life – a bit too nice, maybe. The truth is, my troubles didn't stop after Betty Ford.

In June 1994, hardly more than a month after finishing rehab and being released by the Dodgers, I signed a contract with the San Francisco Giants. That winter brought my IRS woes, which landed me in court. And right in the middle of that mess, I had a drug relapse and failed a test. Major League Baseball suspended me for sixty days, which I served at the start of the 1995 season. Soon after, the Giants decided I was through, and they released me. That's when Bill Goodstein got me to the Yankees.

Everywhere I've been, my battles have come with me. They are a part of me. I know I still have trials ahead, and there's always more soul-searching to do. Once, the thought of living in a constant state of war frightened me. I couldn't handle thinking about it. Now I see how it's exactly that awareness which is going to help me conquer my demons – that and the grace of God. I know I'm at war, and I'm not afraid to say so. For me, it's going to be a fight to the death.

Back when Darryl went into Betty Ford for treatment, I still had an awful lot to learn about recovery. I thought, Oh, he's getting help, and everything's going to be fine. It's all going to be a bed of roses, and we'll walk hand in hand into the sunset... But that's not how it goes.

After he got out of Betty Ford, we moved to Rancho Mirage and Darryl was introduced to a good 12-Step program and began attending meetings regularly. He focused on taking care of himself. I knew I should be happy, but I found myself dealing with more pain, because I still wasn't dealing with the issues I faced as the wife of a recovering alcoholic.

I had heard one such woman tell her story at Betty Ford – or at least I'd been in the room while she was speaking. I had tried to block out what she was saying, because I didn't want to hear anyone say that I had a problem, too. Darryl was the one with the problem, not me...

It took time, but eventually I did come to realize that recovery has as much to do with me as it does with Darryl. I can't spend my life trying to protect or shield him; I've got to see how alcoholism has affected me and deal with that. Once I enrolled in a program for family members of alcoholics, then I began to see that I'm in as much need of recovery as Darryl is, because alcoholism is a disease that affects everyone in contact with it. It's not for nothing that they call it the "family disease."

Recently, I've become close friends with Adele Smithers, whom I call the "Mother of Recovery." Her late husband, R. Brinkley, founded the Smithers Foundation. Adele knows recovery from both ends of the stick – from her own family's experience, and from the people she works with daily. Of course, she knew Darryl from his stay at the Smithers Institute, but it wasn't until his battle with cancer that I first got to know her. Something clicked when we met. She's old enough to be my mom, and she now calls me her adopted daughter; we talk all the time. Having been married to a recovering alcoholic herself, she understands my life and helps me see things in perspective. Because of her I now understand better than ever how important it is that I work a program and see my own need for healing.

The road to recovery never ends; it's one you have to walk down every day, without thinking about what lies ahead. In spite of the hard times, Darryl and I are determined to keep going, no matter what.

Actually, we have no choice. Our children's futures are at

stake, and we're not prepared to gamble with their lives. They mean too much to us.

Jordan was born March 17, 1994, at St. Joseph's Hospital in Orange County. Darryl was at spring training and couldn't be there for the birth, but he managed to get to the hospital later in the day, after Jordan arrived.

But when Jade was born on May 20, 1995, at Eisenhower Hospital in Rancho Mirage, he was there. Jade was our "strike baby." As I like to remind Darryl, "She wouldn't have been conceived if you guys hadn't been on strike." He had taken me to St. Thomas, and that had been the first time we'd really been able to spend together. It made up for not having had a proper honeymoon. And that's where Jade was conceived.

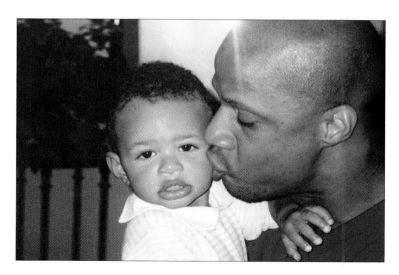

We'd always talked about wanting children, and it worked out well for us: first a boy, and then a girl, and that's it. That's our family.

You said we were going to have five.

Well, I think two is a great number. They're very special kids, so different from each other. Both of them are happy, and so full of energy, which means they keep Charisse and me busy. They're a great challenge.

The way my older children, DJ and Diamond, accept Jordan and Jade makes it very easy and simple for all of us just to be together when those chances come. To me, each of them is so special, so unique.

My kids have taught me a lot about patience. It's clear that the older they get, the more patience I've got to have with them, and that's a big test for me as a parent. But I'm learning how important it is that regardless of what phase the kids go through, you have to go through it with them. You have to learn with them each step of the way, and that requires patience, but most of all love.

Usually, for example, Jordan and Jade don't want to go to bed at night; they're used to staying up late because of our schedule. So I came up with a little game, which they take very seriously. I say, "Okay, since you guys don't want to go to sleep, I'm going to beat you to your bed, and I'm going to sleep there." And they go, "No way!" And then, every night, we race to see if I can get their spot. The rule is, if I win, they have to sleep somewhere else. And they're not too thrilled about that idea! So that's become our good-night ritual. It's my way of getting them to bed.

Our kids are so well-adjusted to the life we live. People say thing like, "Gosh, between baseball and kids, how do you cope?" But I've never thought about it as being a big deal. I've seen so many other women in baseball raise children and manage fine. Thousands of children have grown up this way; it doesn't have to be a hassle.

The beautiful thing is the kids are still young enough to be oblivious to the spotlight we live in. Actually, last year Jordan gave us a little hint that he'd kind of hooked onto something when he started acting out his autograph routine. He'd mimic people asking for autographs, and then pretend to sign his name. So now we have a little game that we play. He comes up and says, "Here. Ask for my autograph, ask for my autograph." So we go, "Okay. Oh, Jordan we love you! You're the best base-ball player. Can we have your autograph?" And then Jordan "signs" for us – or else he copies what Darryl sometimes says when he's with us: "No, I'm busy. I've got my family with me right now." And then Jordan walks off smiling.

Both Jordan and Jade like to go to the games, and they pay attention. Jordan knows the names of all the Yankees' players, and he can mimic each of their batting stances. He loves base-ball – he started pretending to hit a ball with an imaginary bat when he was sixteen months old. And now that he's in Little League, he's always asking to wear Darryl's Yankee jerseys or his batting gloves. He wants to carry his dad's bat and do everything the way Darryl does. Except that Jordan's a righty.

As a kid, I fell in love with baseball. No one put any pressure on me, at least no one in my family ever did. I see a lot of parents today who expect a lot out of their kids. Whether it's soccer or football, basketball or baseball, they want their kids to be out in front, playing and participating in sports. It's good if parents want their kids to play, but I think too many parents pressure their kids to excel, and that takes all the fun out of the game. There's a difference between someone offering encouragement and helping a child channel his or her energies, and a person who puts pressure on a kid to succeed. No one ever drilled into me, "You're going to be this type of player, and this is what I want you to do." And I think that's why I was able to go out and put my heart into the game.

With my kids, especially my two boys, Darryl Jr. and Jordan, I don't ever want to put pressure on them about sports. I've seen players who've had so much pressure put on them by their parents that they just completely crack. They can't handle it. It becomes too much. And that's the last thing I'd want to do to my kids.

They will have to learn to face pressure, though. It will come automatically. Not from Darryl, but just because of their last name. And my feeling is, it's going to be something they'll have to deal with, because both Darryl Jr. and Jordan are gifted with natural athleticism. As parents, it puts a responsibility on us to give our children the assurance that they can be who they are, who God wants them to be. The way I see it, I'd probably actually prefer for Jordan not to be a baseball player. But in the end, that's not for me to decide.

I'd like our children to have an education. Charisse and I want to see them both finish college. If they're interested in getting into sports, college would be a great place for that, too. When

Charisse's brother, Miles, was playing basketball at Arizona, before he got drafted by the Orlando Magic, we used to go to his games. There's something special about college sports. I love watching them, especially basketball and football. But I think college baseball is boring; I guess the idea of an aluminum bat never did much for me...

The kids keep us going. A lot of times, with all the stuff we've been through, I could say, "God, I'm tired." But I look at those kids, and I think, "We've got to do whatever we've got to do for them." Because God has blessed us with two beautiful, healthy children, and that's a gift. We could have had children who were sickly. But we were given two healthy, bright, beautiful kids.

We try our best to instill morals and values in them, to not just let them get away with everything. I want my kids to grow up learning how to do things for themselves, to do chores

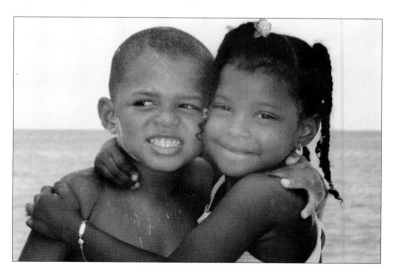

around the house and that kind of thing, so that they don't grow up expecting others to cater to them.

When I think of my children and their futures, I have my worries, too. I worry that people may judge them because of Darryl or give them a hard time because of who their dad is. I want my children to be treated fairly. I want them to have friends who like them for who they are, not because their dad is a professional athlete, or for any other reason. Those are things I worry about, but I think that's just my motherly instinct showing itself; I don't actually think those things will be big problems for my children.

On the other hand, I do have some very real fears: I don't want to see our children destroyed by either cancer or alcoholism, both of which run in the family. Our doctors have already made us aware of what we can do to protect our kids from cancer when they're older, through healthy eating and early detection screening. When it comes to alcoholism, though, that's where they're more at risk – but that's also where our responsibility as parents comes in, to break the cycle for them.

We want our kids to grow up in a healthy environment. Of course, to provide that for them means we have to continue to work on ourselves. Whether it's in helping them get through school, teaching them about cancer, or warning them about the dangers of addiction, it's our job to educate our children. To do that, we have to lead them by example, and that means having the humility to realize that there is always room for growth in us.

Sometimes I think about what life will be like for my children after I'm gone. It makes me realize that it's not important to try to leave a legacy behind for them, at least not a legacy in material things.

I want them to learn about God, that's my concern. And I want them to learn that being "important" has nothing to do with life. That's something my trials have taught me: the world will lift you up and make you important, because the world wants to tear you down. It doesn't matter who you are, that's how it always happens. There's always a stranger with a pad of paper or a TV camera ready to put together a story about you based on things they only half understand. That's what being important does for you.

All anyone really wants out of life is joy. It's a feeling that comes from deep inside; you can't explain how it feels, but you know it when you find it. And joy can be found on earth, but you're going to deal with some very difficult times, too. Joy is the thing I wish most for my children.

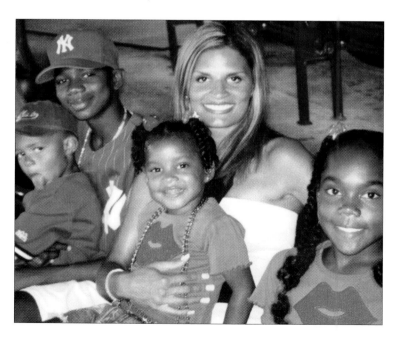

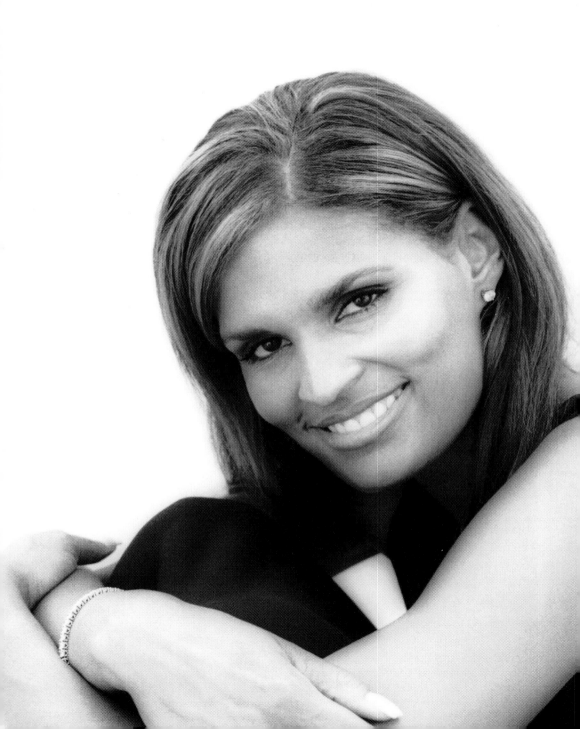

CHAPTER VI

SAINT STRAWBERRY

"It's really all about picking yourself up
and continuing to move forward."

"I look at him and say, emphatically,
'We're not getting a minivan.'"

Every Sunday when we're at home in California, we drive an hour and a half to St. Stephen Baptist Church in La Puente. Charisse joined there in 1993, but for a while after we married she and I attended my mother's church. Eventually, though, not long before Jade was born, she persuaded me to come to St. Stephen with her. Two Sundays later, I joined.

St. Stephen has over four thousand members, I think, but you never feel lost in the congregation. That's partly because there are three different Sunday services, but mostly it's because people make you feel like you belong there, no matter what walk of life you come from.

Our godparents, Ma and Pa Leonard, played a big part in getting me to the church, but they didn't stop there. St. Stephen isn't about warm, fuzzy feelings on Sunday morning. It's about saving lives.

Not long after I'd started coming, Pa Leonard introduced me to Josh. And that's how I got involved with the church's Spiritual 12-Step program.

Josh is the founder and leader of this program, which follows the pattern of Alcoholics Anonymous but includes bible study as well. He's also a recovering alcoholic and drug addict, just like me, except that he's got over fifteen years of sobriety. He introduced me to the program there at St. Stephen and got me started attending meetings. It didn't take long for us to develop a deep level of trust, and I asked him to be my sponsor. Josh has been by my side ever since.

Through Josh I became involved in the church's ministry to the homeless. Every Thursday evening I'm home during the off-season, I go to the church and help pack vans full of food. Then we drive downtown and make our rounds.

We hand out our bags of food to people living on the same streets where I grew up. People tell me, "You'd better watch your back down there," but they forget that I was raised in that atmosphere; I know how to take care of business "down there."

Of course, the reason we go is to try to help as many people as we can. You've got to be heads-up. Sometimes guys will try little stunts like getting a food bag from us at one stop and then meeting us at our next stop and lining up for another. If you ask them about it, they'll tell you, "Yeah, but you know how it is, man. I'm just trying to feed my family..." Once in a while a homeless person will ask for my autograph, but I tell them, "That's not why I'm here," and usually they understand what I mean.

Helping with the food run always leaves me feeling humbled. I can't help thinking that, coming from where I do, I could very easily be in their place. It makes me more thankful, and it helps me keep the issues in my life in perspective. I always come away feeling energized, ready to face life head-on.

Of course, there have been times in my life when I've felt like giving up, or when I've felt so low I couldn't see the point in going on. The winter of '95–'96 was one of those times. My mom died at the end of February, and I basically lost interest in life for a while. It was as if, through her death, the center of the Strawberry universe had burned out. Only when she was gone did I fully realize how much I'd drawn on her seemingly endless supply of inspiration and inner strength to keep me going. Despite Charisse's love and understanding, I wondered how I'd manage without Mom. I guess some of us never outlive our Momma's Boy label...

Adding to my depression after Mom's death was the growing uncertainty about my future in baseball. My one-year contract with the Yankees had expired at the end of the 1995 season. Now it was time for spring training to begin, and my chances of resigning seemed almost zero. True, a few teams around the league contacted my new agent, Eric Grossman, and put out feelers, but nothing that we could feel good about came together. The way things were going, I half expected to sit out for the season.

And then Eric called and left a message, saying he'd been contacted by the St. Paul Saints, an independent team in the Northern

League whose principal owner is Marv Goldklang, who also happens to be a limited partner with the Yankees. His partners in the Saints include the comedian Bill Murray and Mike Veeck, son of the famous Bill Veeck. Marv, as it turned out, was very interested in seeing me in a Saints uniform. I'd never heard of the Northern League, let alone the St. Paul Saints, and my immediate reaction, voiced to Charisse, was, "I'm not playing in *that*."

Actually, it was more along the lines of "I'm not going. I'll retire. I'll quit. I don't want to play anymore..." Darryl was pretty frustrated with baseball, and tired of having to prove himself everywhere we went. In the end, though, the bottom line remained unchanged: he needed a job, and no major league team seemed willing to offer him one. So by mid-March, when it looked like nothing else was going to pan out, we made the decision to give St. Paul a shot. Through Eric, we struck a deal: Darryl would earn $2000 a month and could leave at any time if he chose to sign with a major league team – and Marv Goldklang had taken up Darryl's cause as a kind of personal crusade.

Six weeks later, at the beginning of May, we packed our bags, took the kids, and got on a plane to St. Paul.

We arrive in Minnesota and load our luggage into a rented minivan at the airport. Darryl gets behind the wheel and drives. The first thing I know, he's saying to me, "This thing handles nicely. We should get one of these."

I think, This is bizarre. We're out in the middle of nowhere, heading into the unknown, and he's talking about buying a minivan. I look at him and say, emphatically, "We're not getting a minivan."

Within days of our arrival in St. Paul, the team leaves for a pre-season road trip. Darryl, because he's still Darryl – even if no one in the big leagues thinks so anymore – isn't required to ride the team bus with the other players. Most are young, single guys, but we've got kids, and there's no way I'm staying behind in some strange apartment with them. So we get back into the minivan and tag along behind the bus, past fields full of cows and on into uncharted territory, en route to Duluth. Watching Darryl, I imagine he has a cartoon thought-bubble floating over his head. It reads: "What am I *doing?* I'm on a road trip, with my wife and kids. And I'm driving a minivan…"

Back in 1983, when the Mets had made me the top pick in the first round of the draft, it never once occurred to me that the day might come when I wouldn't be playing in "The Show." Even if the thought had crossed my mind, the people around me wouldn't have allowed me to believe it for a minute. After all, in their eyes I was set to become the "black Ted Williams" (my high school coach once used that phrase referring to me in conversation, and the media picked it up), and although I tried not to get carried away by other people's expectations, I knew that if I used my talent to my advantage, I would go far in the major leagues.

Of course back then I was just a naïve kid from Crenshaw High who lived and breathed baseball, but knew next to nothing about what it takes to stay alive. I certainly didn't have any idea what I was in for.

We won the city basketball championship my senior year of high school and then went to Oakland for the state tournament, but we didn't make it out of the first round. So I got back home and managed to make it to one day of baseball practice before the season started two days later. That first game, at least fifty people showed up – to see me. I asked my coach, "What's all this about?" and he said he'd been getting a lot of calls about me from major league scouts. "He's playing basketball right now. Just hope he doesn't hurt himself," he'd told them. So at our first game, fifty or so scouts show up, as well as TV reporters and everything.

The things they said about me: "He believes in himself." "There's no fear in him when he's on the field." "This kid's got a frame that's going to develop, and he's going to be a tremendous home run hitter." I didn't know where they pulled half that stuff from, but that's what they were saying.

Well, my season started off horribly; blame it on basketball, I guess. But then, after about five games, I started playing like I was possessed. I was winning games, hitting grand slams, knocking the ball out of the park. Everything seemed to come together all at once. I wasn't thinking about scouts or anything like that. It was all about winning, right now.

The year before, my junior year, we'd made it to the city championship at Dodger Stadium, but we'd lost to some guy called John Elway, who was pitching for Grenada Hills. So my senior year, I wanted us to get back and win it.

We got back, all right, but again we fell short of the championship. Still, I was rewarded: my last at-bat as a high school kid, I hit a home run in Dodger Stadium. That sealed my fate. All the scouts said the same thing: "That's it! He's the number-one draft pick."

How come? I asked myself. How come, out of all the great baseball players my age across the country, I'm the one people are predicting will be selected first in the draft — me, a skinny kid out of Crenshaw High... I'd always hoped my baseball dreams would one day come true, but this was way past my imagination.

The rest is history. I became a Met in 1980 and started playing rookie ball with the farm team in Kingsport, Tennessee, and had to face the reality of being away from home for the first time in my life. The next season, I started A ball in Lynchburg, Virginia. Then, in 1982, I played with the Double-A team in Jackson, Mississippi, and finished the season by playing Triple-A in Tidewater. I started the 1983 season there in Virginia, but on May 5 I was at the plate in Shea Stadium, facing Cincinnati's Mario Soto for my first major league at-bat — which also happened to coincide with my first major league strikeout. That first game, I came to bat four times. I struck out my first three chances, then popped out my last time up.

I wound up going 0–11 before getting my first hit in the majors. Everyone on the team kept saying, "Relax. You'll be fine. Just relax and hang in there." Then on May 16, in my twenty-seventh at-bat, I hit my first big-league home run, and went on to win the Rookie of the Year Award. And the rest is also history.

Of course, even as I was coming up through the Mets' farm system, I was learning that professional baseball is like any other business: the bottom line is the bottom line. With the exception of a few very special individuals, most people didn't really care about me as a person. They cared about my numbers: batting average, RBIs, home runs, etc. That's how they measured my worth. Of course, that's good business sense, but when you begin to realize that to many people you're a piece of meat, a machine, well, it helps you rub the stars from your eyes.

As long as you're a success story, people want to be along for the ride. They'll party with you and pass you a drink, slap your back and say, "Yeah, that's my buddy Darryl!" But once things start slipping, once you show weakness and have a downfall or two, then these same people slink away, and you hear them say, "Hmm, I always wondered what was wrong with him." Pretty soon, when you realize that the people around you are only there to try to soak up a bit of the "glory" that supposedly surrounds you, you start asking yourself, "What's the point?" And that's how you open the door for destructive forces to enter your life. You kick your nightlife into high gear as a way to drown everything out. Worse, you start to hate yourself. Before you know it, you're in big trouble, caught in a cycle that takes years to break.

I guess, in a way, that explains at least part of the reason why a guy who "everyone" predicted would one day be a Hall of Fame shoo-in winds up financially strapped and thankful for a job opportunity with an independent-league team in Minnesota. It goes a long way to explain why on May 31, 1996, I found myself in a minivan with my wife and kids, driving over a hundred and fifty miles to a ballgame against a team called the Duluth-Superior Dukes.

It was all so new, so different. We pulled into Duluth – the fog coming in off Lake Superior and the confusing one-way streets reminded us of San Francisco – and checked in at the Holiday Inn. Compared with what we were used to, the place was a dump – no adjoining room for the kids or anything. I took one look and said, "Wow." But that's all there was to be said.

The Duluth stadium was freezing (I found myself remembering Darryl's games in Candlestick Park back in the summer of 1994, when he'd played for the San Francisco Giants). If I remember rightly, the Saints played three games against the Dukes. One was rained out, but Darryl hit three home runs in the course of the other two – a sign of things to come.

Back at the Saints' Midway Stadium in St. Paul, the fans welcomed Darryl enthusiastically. They cheered each time he stepped to the plate, and with increasing frequency Darryl rewarded them by hitting tape-measure home runs. His swing was loose, and the ball just seemed to explode off his bat as it left the stadium. With each game it seemed he was recapturing the love for the game that had propelled him into pro ball to begin with, and there was something infectious about that. After all, this was a whole different kind of baseball.

Mike Veeck, who runs the Saints, deserves credit for bringing out the fun in baseball in ways we'd never seen before. He's best known for the worst night of his professional life, "Disco Demolition Night," a baseball promotion-turned-nightmare he orchestrated for his father's Chicago White Sox back in the seventies. But that's not what he's associated with in St. Paul.

Thanks to Mike, games at Midway Stadium are more than just games, they're events, with give-aways and contests. "Win a night to sit and watch the game from the Jacuzzi overlooking right field" – that kind of thing. Between innings, fans are invited onto the field for activities like Dizzy Bat races (the basic idea: stand a baseball bat vertically and plaster your nose to its end, spin yourself around as fast as you can until someone yells "Go!" and then see if you can run the base path from first to second in something resembling a straight line. Nothing to it, really…) or "sumo wrestling," which involves two fans dressed up in inflatable sumo suits trying desperately to deck each other while the stadium PA system blares a song with the catchy line, "It's kung-fu fighting!"

Like I said, we were experiencing a whole new approach to baseball. When Jade turned one year old, they wished her a happy birthday over the loudspeakers at the game. She and Jordan, who was two, would sit in the stands with me every night, and they paid close attention when their daddy got up to bat.

They weren't the only ones.

Compared to our high-profile life in New York, being in St. Paul was a bit like falling down Alice's rabbit hole and landing in Wonderland. But it wasn't as if the media had altogether forgotten Darryl. Nor had the professional scouts, who appeared once Darryl's home run numbers started piling up. During June several offers from major league teams came our way, with the Cincinnati Reds showing perhaps the most serious interest. Then on the evening of July 3, during a 12–0 blowout of the Sioux Falls Canaries, Darryl hit his eighteenth home run as a

Saint to set a new franchise record. During the fourth inning, manager Marty Scott waved Darryl in from right field to give him the news: The Yankees had called, and they wanted him back – right away.

Darryl signed the one-year deal and boarded a flight to Columbus, Ohio, where he was slated to play a few games with the Yankees' Triple-A team, that same night.

Ideally, I would have liked to have stayed for the Independence Day game in St. Paul. It would have been a chance to say good-bye to the fans, to let them know how much they'd given me, even if they hadn't realized it. But that wasn't meant to be. Charisse would have to step up to the plate for me the next night and say "thank you" and "good-bye" for both of us. About the only thing I had time for was to grab a couple of my bats and get everyone in the clubhouse to sign them for me, as mementos. Then I was out of there, starting the first leg of my journey back to New York.

As I settled in my seat for the flight to Columbus, my mind raced as I thought about getting back to the Yankees. But at the same time I couldn't help going back over the two months I'd spent in Saints uniform and realizing, once again, just how much I had to be thankful for.

When you've played your whole career in the majors, you have to swallow a lot of pride to accept a job at minor league level. Going to St. Paul, that was something I had to deal with, but I also knew I could count myself lucky to be playing at all. That's what

I tried to tell myself, but I guess some self-pity must have still been clinging to me, because it took Dave Stevens to make me see just how lucky I was – and am.

I met Dave the first day of spring training, on the field at Midway Stadium. Dave was different than the other guys on the field, in more ways than one. The most obvious difference was his lack of legs; they were simply missing. But Dave knew how to hustle. He'd "run" around the outfield, pulling himself with his hands and arms, and catch fly balls with the team. His upper body was strong, and he could hit the ball quite well – an added bonus was his tiny strike zone.

Dave inspired me. Here was a guy who wanted so badly to work out with a baseball team that he pestered Saints' management into letting him take part in spring training. "The little guy," as I dubbed him, didn't know the meaning of the word "disability," but he sure understood the term "heart." Next to the problems he faced each and every day, what did I have to worry about?

One of my happiest moments as a Saint came during an exhibition game in Madison, Wisconsin, when Marty Scott agreed to let Dave take my at-bat in the ninth inning. Even though Dave struck out, it made me glad to see my friend at the plate, playing for real. When our season started and he headed back to Connecticut and his job with ESPN, I missed him.

Playing in St. Paul was like playing Little League all over again – and I don't mean that as a slur against Northern League pitchers. Not since my childhood had playing ball been so much fun. I learned to relax again, to enjoy my God-given talents, doing what I do best, fully supported and encouraged by people like Mike Veeck and Marv Goldklang, who love baseball for its beauty.

But maybe the best part about being in St. Paul was that it allowed me, Charisse, Jordan, and Jade to be the little Strawberry family we really are. We were still coming to terms with losing my mom and with the death of Bill, and St. Paul gave us a chance to catch our breath. Sure, the spotlight followed me west to Minnesota, but with nowhere near the wattage I'd known in New York. For the first time in years I felt we could lead at least a semi-normal life as a family, and we did our best to enjoy that privilege while it lasted. It wouldn't last for ever, I knew. Once I got my game in focus, I felt sure we'd be leaving St. Paul before too long.

They say that good things come to those who wait. And they did – thanks to Mr. Steinbrenner. He defied his critics and offered me the job that gave me a chance to help the Yankees get to and win the 1996 World Series. More important, for the Strawberry family at least, it opened a new window for us and gave us a chance to start all over again.

And so I left Minnesota, feeling energized, ready to face life head-on.

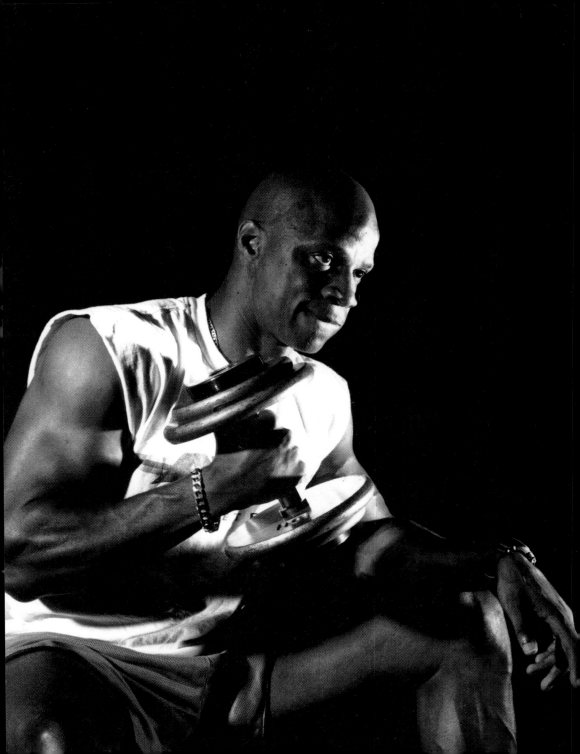

CHAPTER VII

LONG ROAD HOME

"I was dreaming of cheesecake..."

"I'd never been to the stadium without him either
in the game or by my side, and it just felt strange."

After Darryl's successful surgery on October 3, 1998, we anticipated a speedy recovery. He wouldn't have to stay in the hospital much more than a week, the doctors told us. That was good news. We were looking forward to going home and being together as a family again.

Then an infection developed in Darryl's colon, which brought on flu-like symptoms: fever, nausea, dizzy spells. It's not unusual for this to happen after colon surgery, and there was no reason for alarm. But now we were looking at a full two weeks before Darryl would be able to come home. For me, it was a mentally tough situation, having to watch him put up with the pain and being helpless to do anything about it.

Darryl knew that several months of chemotherapy still lay ahead, and he wanted to get home as soon as possible so he could get on with it. The infection was a setback, and it really frustrated him. He did his best not to show it, particularly in front of visitors or media people, but he couldn't hide it from me.

As a couple, we'd never been so much in the public eye before. Reporters were hanging out around the hospital, hoping for any news: "How's Darryl doing? Is he hungry?" "Yeah," I told them, "he says he wants cheesecake." That got a laugh, but it was an answer I'd end up eating out – literally. Whenever I was home with the kids, the reporters would wait outside our house until we came out again. After one paper ran a photo of my kids walking down the stairs from our house with a friend of ours (the caption: "Family Pal: A friend of Darryl & Charisse Strawberry picks up their kids for a play date"), I decided it was getting ridiculous. After that, we loaded the kids into the car before leaving the garage.

Meanwhile, all day long teammates, coaches, and friends were coming in and out of Darryl's hospital room. He didn't want to look depressed or unhappy with them around. So by the time I would get to his room in the afternoon, he would be pretty worn out, and his nerves raw. Then, since I'm his wife and the closest person to him in the world, he'd take his frustrations out on me. He was climbing the walls, and I understood.

Going into surgery, I was already twenty pounds under my playing weight of 225. By the time I was released from the hospital,

I was down to 186. So even though I knew my outlook was as good as I could hope for, I still had to deal with feeling really helpless during those two weeks in Columbia-Presbyterian. They kept me catheterized and in bed for a while after the surgery. Then, after I was allowed to start walking a bit, I had to push my IV stand around with me everywhere I went. That side of things was no fun, and Charisse showed her patience once again, letting me vent my frustrations.

Yet even though I couldn't wait to get out of the hospital and really start to recover, I had an overwhelming feeling of gratefulness inside of me. God had protected me so far, and I felt certain he'd see me through.

I knew how lucky I was that my cancer had been discovered at such an early stage of development. The surgeons had removed thirty-six lymph nodes from the area around the tumor, and their tests showed that the cancer had only infected one of these nodes, one that had been located right on top of the tumor. They told me this was a good sign: there was no indication the disease had spread anywhere else.

Then there were the patients in the ward around me. Many of them were suffering conditions far worse than mine. Some of them were dying. One patient passed away in a room just down the hall from me. Another young girl – she was twenty-two, I think – had just gone through major brain surgery. Even though I went through periods of feeling helpless, I knew I was going to recover. But for many of the people around me, their chances weren't nearly as good as mine.

Throughout my stay in the hospital, friends were by my side. I was surrounded by people who cared about me, people who wanted the best for me, and even though when you're trying to get your strength back after a big surgery it can be wearing to have a lot of people around, I really appreciated knowing how much everyone cared. Each day, literally hundreds of letters and cards arrived from all over the country, and even some from abroad – some from fans, some from sworn Yankee adversaries. But all of them wanted to let me know their thoughts were with me: "Get well soon..." "We're praying for you..." "We miss you. Get back in the game..."

Columbia-Presbyterian has a ward for children suffering from cancer, and when they heard I was in the hospital, they sent me some of the most special letters I received during those two weeks. When I thought about those kids facing cancer just as their lives were beginning, it made me feel very humble. They tried to reach out to me, because they knew their pain was my pain. They knew that as cancer patients we all belonged to the same family.

For me, I can't think of anything worse than knowing a kid is suffering with cancer. A kid hasn't had a chance to find out what life is or to fulfill dreams. I know the pain cancer causes, and that makes it all the more devastating to think of a child having to deal with this disease. And yet more than anything or anyone, it was those children who made me understand that I had better be grateful for having survived so far. They were survivors – they believed they could beat their disease – and when you get that attitude from a kid, it forces you to believe in your own heart.

Three days after Darryl's tumor was removed, the Yankees faced the Cleveland Indians for Game 1 of the American League

Championship Series. I got a call from the Yankees' front office, and they said, "Mr. Steinbrenner wants you to throw out the first pitch." Right away I thought of Darryl back in his room at the hospital, and I told them, "Uh, I don't really want to do that." They persisted: "Well, George really, really wants you to." I said I'd talk it over with Darryl.

Darryl didn't take long to respond when I told him. "Well," he said, "if the boss wants you to do it, then you should do it." So that was it. "Okay, Darryl," I said.

Tuesday night, October 6, I dressed to go to the game, pinning a little gold guardian angel brooch on the lapel of my gray suit. Then I took Jordan and Jade over to the hospital to see their dad before we headed for the stadium. The last thing Darryl said to me was, "Don't embarrass me. Throw a strike."

I'd never been to the stadium without him either in the game or by my side, and it just felt strange. My children noticed it too.

I wasn't prepared to face the media, but when we arrived the team representatives asked me if I could field a few questions. I said, "How many?" They assured me, "Just a few." So they took me to a press conference room – I think it was the same room the team uses for post-game interviews – and it seemed there were a hundred reporters in there, with cameras and lights. And I had to go up and sit in front of them all, with a big American League Series banner in back of me. There was a woman sitting on a stool next to me who was fielding the questions and repeating them to me, and I tried to answer as best I could while everyone scribbled notes. I did my best to conduct myself with poise and dignity, but I was just glad when the session was over.

I took the kids with me down to the dugout. Jordan cried and screamed. The players tried to help. Derek Jeter came over and tried to calm him down, but Jordan wasn't having it: "My daddy's not here!" He didn't want to go with me onto the field. Jade, on the other hand, couldn't figure out why we were waiting. "Come on, Mommy!" she kept saying.

At the last minute, they gave me Darryl's jersey and asked me to wear it. So I had to take my coat off and put the jersey on. I was nervous. So nervous I was shaking all over. I felt cold. Then David Cone, who's been a close friend of Darryl's since their days together with the Mets, walked me and the kids out onto the grass in front of the mound…

The stadium is shaking, or is it just me? My ears tell me it's not. The stands are jam-packed with fans, all of them on their feet, screaming and yelling as Darryl's picture comes up on the big screen. I can't really see anything. David hands me the ball, and I know Joe Girardi is behind the plate waiting for my throw – but I can't see him. I'm so choked up, and I can't stop the tears. Jordan and Jade are hanging onto me. I throw the ball. It makes a weak arch and lands in the dirt in front of the plate…

The Yankee players took the field wearing Darryl's number, 39, embroidered on their hats; they'd started that for Game 3 of the Division Series against Texas. It touched me to see their concern for Darryl, and later, when I learned that players from other teams in the playoffs were pencilling "39" in white on their hats as well, it was hard to know what to say in response.

As the game got underway, I took Jade and Jordan down to the playroom so they could be with their friends. Then Ma Leonard and I headed for our seats in the players' family section. It was comforting to be surrounded by our friends, the wives and children of Darryl's teammates. Everybody was so nice, and they were all wearing Darryl's number on pinstriped buttons. They hugged us and told us how much they were thinking of us. Kim Girardi, Joe's wife, gave me a box of strawberries dipped in chocolate with "39" on them. (Later, she had gold strawberry-shaped pins made, with "39" and a cross in their centers, and the players' wives wore them at the games we missed, in honor of me and of Darryl.) Around the stadium, fans were holding signs, messages for Darryl: things like "Strawberry fields forever" and "Get well, Straw." Instead of the usual "K" signs, they hung up pictures of strawberries whenever David got a strikeout. Darryl was on everyone's mind.

But suddenly all I wanted to do was cry. I felt so out of place, so uncomfortable. Mr. Steinbrenner had invited me to watch the game from his suite, and I went by to see him. But I couldn't stay long; I just didn't want to be there anymore. I had to get back to Darryl. I told Ma Leonard, "I've got to go." So we picked up the kids and left.

Darryl was awake when we got back to the hospital. He was watching the game. "You threw like a girl," he said. A while later, my father called from California. He said the same thing…

Going into the hospital, I knew my season was over. It felt good to watch the team get that first win, 7–2, over Cleveland, and I knew we'd take care of business. But as for me, I concentrated on trying to have a good attitude toward my situation. Once I knew it was cancer I was dealing with, I said to myself, "Hey, let's get this taken care of, just get on with it." Even though it was going to be a long road back, at least that was better than how it had been before, when we hadn't known what was wrong with me. Still, being in the hospital for two weeks – it was unbelievable.

I think it was because he sneaked in a cookie. He wasn't supposed to eat. That's probably why he got that infection in his colon.

Yeah, two weeks without eating solid foods. They give you Jell-O and broth and water.

He was a big complainer.

I was like, "Bring on the real food." I was dreaming of cheese-cake, eating cheesecake in my sleep.

And because of what I'd told the media, people kept sending me cheesecakes for Darryl. I lost count of the cheesecakes mailed to me. They were all over our house, and Ma Leonard, my grandmother, and I ate them over coffee until we didn't want to look at another slice. We gave them away to nurses at the hospital, and still bakeries all over New York kept sending

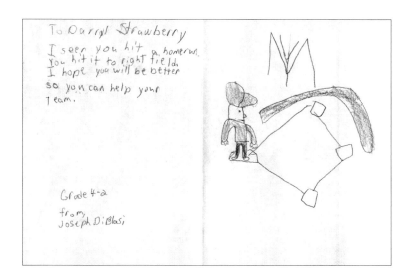

To Darryl Strawberry
I seen you hit a homerun.
You hit it to right field.
I hope you will be better
so you can help your
Team.

Grade 4-2

from
Joseph DiBlasi

cheesecakes. Maybe I should have done a "hold the cheese-cakes" press conference…

For me, the most frustrating thing was losing all that weight. As an athlete, that was especially tough, because everything about my career depends on my physical strength and health. I know Charisse put up with a lot from me, and I'll always be grateful to her for the understanding and care she showed me during those difficult days at Columbia-Presbyterian. She proved once more that she is the backbone of our family.

And then, finally, the big day came. Actually, it was more like a big moment. Before Darryl could be released, he had to meet the standard requirement for patients who've been through colon surgery: he had to pass gas. Normally in our household, that's an annoying habit, but that day we cheered.

It meant everything was in working order – the IV could come out, and Darryl could start eating small portions of solids. Not long after, on October 16, he was discharged and we headed for our home in Fort Lee.

I made it home in time to watch Game 1 of the World Series, Yankees against the San Diego Padres, on Saturday, October 17. There'd been rumors in the press that I might be at the stadium to throw out the first pitch, but I was in no condition to do that. Charisse and I watched the Fox broadcast on our living room TV.

That was hard, sitting there watching the team. In a way, it might have been harder for me than for Darryl. I thought he deserved to be there.

I'd had such a good season, and I'd fully expected to be part of what the team was trying to accomplish. So, yeah, sitting at home was really a test. But at the same time, that's life – things happen.

We watched the entire Series together in front of the TV. I could see Darryl feeding off the energy of the team. The players kept calling the house to talk to us and encourage us to hang tough. They were going to win for Darryl, they told us.

When third baseman Scott Brosius hit his three-run shot over Qualcomm Stadium's center field wall to put the Yankees up 5–3 in Game 3, Darryl went nuts. He jumped off the couch. I was like, "Oh, my God!" I was worried he'd tear the staples out of his stomach.

It was just the excitement of it. I felt I was there. Even though I wasn't in the dugout in uniform, my spirit was there with the guys.

When Mariano Rivera got that final out in the ninth inning of Game 4 and all the Yankees piled on top of each other in celebration, I cried as I hugged Darryl. "Girl, what're you crying for?" he wanted to know, and I didn't know what to tell him. My emotions were mixed: the team had won, but Darryl hadn't been there. It was a special moment, a very sweet moment, but it would have been still sweeter if he had played.

Now it was all over but the shouting. And in the locker room after the game, players drenched in Dom Perignon took care of that, chanting "Straw Man! Straw Man!" Then our phone rang, and Derek Jeter was on the line, with the rest of the team right there. No one had anything very coherent to say, but everyone wanted us to be part of the celebration.

That was Wednesday night, October 21. Earlier that day, Darryl and I had made our first public appearance since his surgery. We were at the Modell's Sporting Goods store on 42nd Street to unveil a special Yankee towel with Darryl's name and number on it, which was going on sale to help raise money for cancer research. We knew fans would be happy to see Darryl, but I don't think we were quite prepared for how wildly excited they were. It was beautiful.

Two days later, on Friday, the Yankees' victory parade lined up outside the stadium. Darryl's doctors had told us it was okay for him to take part, but that we should head home the minute Darryl felt worn out. We went to the locker room at the stadium, and everyone wanted to hug Darryl and tell him how they'd missed him. Then we got into the parade car and joined the fun, though we had to miss the ceremony outside City Hall.

I was exhausted, but it was an unbelievable feeling riding down the "Canyon of Heroes" and hearing all of New York cheering us on. As I waved to the crowd, the thought never crossed my mind that I might be waving good-bye to baseball. I was already thinking about my next step: getting to California and starting chemotherapy. That was my focus, finding my way back to being strong enough to play again.

By the end of October we were packed and ready to leave for Rancho Mirage. The kids had already flown out with Nana and my uncle Rodney, who'd come out to help us pack up the house, a week or so before Darryl and I left, so the five-hour flight to LA was a quiet one, with time to think about the future. A lot of anxiety and work still lay ahead; that was obvious to us. But we'd survived so much already, even in just a couple weeks, that neither of us felt – not even for a moment – that we wouldn't make it through. Again and again we reminded each other not to look too far ahead, and to take life as it comes.

A note that is meant for all of you

especially to say "many thanks for all you've done

in such a thoughtful way."

Thank you for the many prayers, cards, visits, and

beautiful gifts that were sent our way.

It meant the world to Darryl and our family

as we struggled through this challenge brought before us.

Darryl is now doing well and on the road to

a successful recovery. We thank God for our many

wonderful friends and acquaintances like you.

God Bless You All

Darryl and Charisse Strawberry

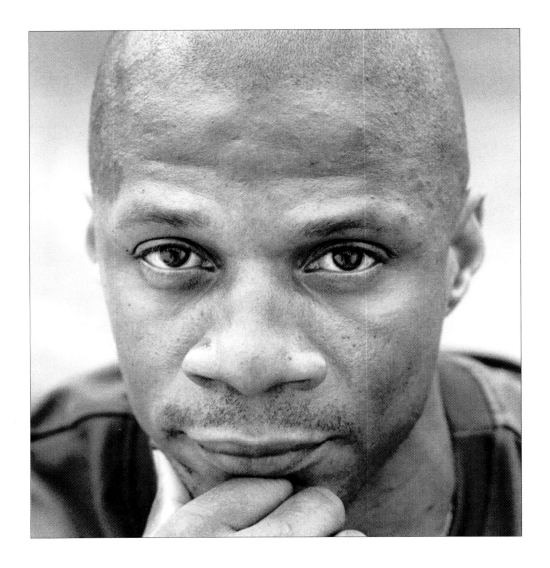

CHAPTER VIII

GAME FACE

•

"We could walk along the beach
or just sit in the shade and watch the
people walking their dogs."

"Nana stayed at our house, and we ate potatoes."

Tick tock, tick tock, tick tock... Like the crocodile that swallowed the alarm clock in *Peter Pan,* my recovery from cancer was eating away at my time. It was November already. February would come around soon enough – and that's when spring training starts. Luckily for me, I'd learned many years before what hard work and dedication are all about...

I got kicked off the baseball team my junior year in high school. I was taking too much for granted and not putting enough effort into my game, and the coach didn't like what he was seeing. He knew I had talent – everyone knew that – but he wanted to send me a message that talent alone doesn't cut it. In the big leagues, everyone's got talent; it's the player with discipline who comes through as the real winner.

Once school was out, I spent that whole summer playing ball, and I really matured in a lot of ways. I learned to accept the coaches' instructions without always thinking I knew better. I realized that I could turn around – I could be not only a good ball player but somebody who was teachable, and I think that was the most important lesson I learned. The next spring, when baseball tryouts came along at Crenshaw High, I showed up with a whole new attitude, ready to play and ready to hustle.

Really, it was just a matter of going back to what Mr. Mosely had taught me in my younger years. My oldest brother, Michael, played for him in the Babe Ruth League and kept telling his coach, "I have a kid brother who's going to be a pretty good ball player." So one day Mr. Mosely came over to our house and told me he wanted to start working with me on my game. He saw from the start that I had the desire to play, even if I didn't always remember that myself. Sometimes he'd have to come over and pull me out of bed to get me to go and work out, and he kept after me, encouraging me to work hard and be tough on myself. He saw something in me that I didn't see in myself and that no one else had noticed yet. I was a skinny kid with an afro, lazy for the most part, and not really sure where I wanted to go in life. But he believed I was going to be a star at the major league level, and so he pushed me. He refused to let me go. He was my first father figure, a man who helped me understand that I could be somebody if I put my mind to it...

And now it was November 1998. I knew I was going to need all the determination and discipline I could come up with if I was going to make it through the winter and be ready to join the team in Tampa. Spring training was only three-and-a-half months away.

Back in Rancho Mirage, we got the kids settled back at their preschool, and then we lined up Darryl's chemotherapy and got ready for that adventure. Our first plan was to have a nurse come in and administer the chemo at our house. But when we visited the Comprehensive Cancer Center in Palm Springs and met the oncologist recommended to us, Dr. Sanford Kempin, Darryl decided to go there regularly.

Three weeks after our return to California his treatment began. For the first four days they gave him intravenous injections of Leucovorin, to make his cells receptive to the chemo. It took about thirty minutes for all the medication to enter his bloodstream. After those four days of intensive treatment, he had to return once every week so that Dr. Kempin could administer the chemotherapy.

They hook you up to an IV, which is just like any other IV, except that the medicine they're putting into your body is actually poison. That's what chemotherapy is: poison that kills cancerous cells. But of course it has an effect on healthy cells, too.

We were prepared for the usual side effects – fatigue, nausea, diarrhea – but they never came. He just never got sick; it was like he was Superman or something.

For the first few weeks I went with Darryl to the Cancer

Center to chemo sessions. Those times together became our "chemo dates." We'd pick up a nice healthy lunch from the cafeteria and eat it in our room, a suite overlooking the mountains. It was almost relaxing, sitting there and carrying on a conversation or watching TV while the nurses and doctors got the chemo pumping into Darryl's arm. When it was over, we'd go home and Darryl would take a nap before going to the gym to work out. Actually, sometimes he wouldn't even bother with a nap and would go straight to the gym. We kept up that pattern for the first several weeks.

The doctors were impressed by the speed of my recovery. Before my operation back in New York, the surgeon, Dr. Todd, had said he wished every patient had an abdomen like mine; he called it a "six pack." Because I was in such good shape, it made it easier for them to cut through my muscle tissue. It also helped me recover well. Within about two months, the incision had healed over. Sometimes I'd look down at it and just kind of go, "Wow!" I guess I had to get used to that scar being there. Charisse was always telling me to stop touching it, but I wasn't even aware that that's what I was doing. Nana finally told her, "Don't worry, that's just his therapy. Leave him alone."

Now that my surgery was behind me and my chemotherapy was underway, I felt that nothing could stop me from getting back in shape in time for spring training. I started slowly at first – I didn't want to hurt myself and screw things up – but pretty soon I was working out every day, and I could feel my muscles start to build once more. It was mostly a matter of trying not to get ahead of myself, just sticking to what I needed to achieve each day.

And whenever I needed a bit of encouragement, I could always find it in one of the countless letters that arrived each day. Sometimes what I read brought me up short and made me realize that even my toughest moments could be used to help someone else, like the writer of the following letter.

November 24, 1998

Mr. Darryl Strawberry
C/O Yankee Stadium
Bronx, New York

Dear Darryl:

I realize that you must get tons of letters from people on a daily basis but I wanted to write to tell you how you have changed my life as well as that of my family.

Since the news reported that you had Colon Cancer on October 1st I found myself following your updates and a strong interest developed in me regarding your symptoms. I became concerned because whenever I had the news on and you were mentioned along with the symptoms I found my self saying "I have that symptom".

To make a long story short, because of the press given your diagnosis, I went to my doctor on October 14th and after a series of test was diagnosed with colon cancer on October 19th. The surgery was performed on October 23rd and I have since been told that all the cancer was removed and I should look forward to a full recovery.

I believe that if it weren't for you I would have put off going to the doctor and who knows when it would have been detected. You and I have traveled down the same road regarding the colon cancer, family emotions, personal emotions and the pain involved in recovery. Because of this I feel a bond and want you to know if ever I can return the favor that you did for me and my family all you have to do is ask.

Just saying "Thank You" doesn't seem enough for someone who probably saved my life but I hope you find some comfort in knowing how much you have impacted my life, and most important, the life of my family.

Sincerely,

Kirk C. Mackey

We celebrated our fifth wedding anniversary on December 3, and for the first time since Darryl's surgery we really spent time alone, just the two of us. We left the kids with Nana and my uncle Rodney and took off for the weekend to Santa Barbara, where we stayed in a little villa right on the beach. Darryl behaved very out of character: when we arrived he had a dozen roses and a fruit platter waiting for me in the room. "See, I'm romantic," he told me. Sure, Darryl, I thought to myself...

That was a beautiful weekend. We were together, doing nothing. Santa Barbara was a quiet place to be. We could stroll along the beach or just sit in the shade and watch the people walking their dogs. People recognized us, but it was no big deal. He took me to dinner and a movie, and I dragged him to the mall. And we talked.

Times like that are few and far between for us, especially during the off-season, when everything centers around Darryl being ready for spring training. In all our years together, there's never been an off-season where he hasn't felt the pressure to push himself. We've never been able to coast or just kick back with the kids. The pressure just doesn't go away. Somehow Darryl always has to be proving something to someone, always going to this or that mini-camp to work out and show that he can perform. At least that's how it seems from my perspective.

For us, the off-season is over before it starts. I've developed my own way of gauging our time at home: If the team makes it to the post-season, we get back to California at the end of October, and then it's Thanksgiving and after that our anniversary,

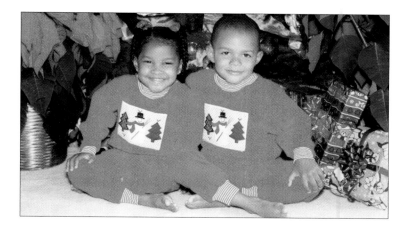

followed by Christmas. Once we hit my birthday in January, that's when I know it's time to start packing up the house again, because three weeks later we leave for Tampa. (And of course after that it's only weeks before we're in New Jersey.) Really, when you stop to add it up, we don't spend a lot of time at home.

Fighting cancer, you realize that life can be short. So we've learned, and we're continuing to learn, that we have to make sure the time we do spend together is quality time.

Everything was going well. Chemotherapy wasn't giving me any problems, and I was starting to bulk up again through my work-outs. Then one morning in early January, I woke up and things were different…

"Charisse, something's wrong. My stomach hurts." From the look on his face, I know something's not right, and he refuses to get out of bed. I come in to check on him every so often, and to remind him to keep taking fluids. He lies there for hours. Then I come in and find him on his hands and knees on the bed. "I'm in a lot of pain," he tells me. "I don't know what's wrong, if it's flu, or what." I say, "Let's call your oncologist," and I get on the line with Dr. Kempin. He listens, then asks me to bring Darryl over to the Center…

It's a good thing we went, because the doctors discovered that a buildup of scar tissue from the surgery had literally formed knots around Darryl's intestine, almost completely blocking it. That explained his stomach pain.

They put a tube up Darryl's nose and down his throat to try to alleviate the pressure on his intestine. I think the doctors hoped the knots would untangle of their own accord once they inserted that tube, but it didn't work. Dr. Kempin ordered some x-rays, then conferred with Dr. Janet Ihde, a surgeon, to get her opinion. She concluded that we had no choice but for Darryl to go back into surgery; if they didn't operate to remove the scar tissue, there was a risk of gangrene setting in, which would then mean having to remove more intestine.

That was the last thing we wanted to hear. At that point Darryl and I were both feeling overly strained. I remember thinking, How do I deal with this? All I could say was, "God, please help me through. Please help us through this one, too." Because you just don't know what can happen; there are too many things that can go wrong.

There was a lot of back and forth with Darryl's doctors in New York, but they too agreed that surgery was the only alternative. Dr. LaPook told me not to worry, that Dr. Ihde was a very competent surgeon and knew what she was doing. So that same night, at eleven o'clock, she and her team performed the operation. We kept the whole thing under wraps, because I just knew I couldn't deal with the press again. The thought of that made me real panicky.

They cut me open again right along the same scar as where they'd first gone in. Luckily they didn't have to make such a big incision, more like half the length of the first one. It only took about forty-five minutes for Dr. Ihde to remove the knots that had tangled themselves around my colon, and to do whatever it was she had to do to help lessen the chance of a lot of scar tissue redeveloping.

I knew that scar tissue problems were common after colon surgery, and Dr. Ihde assured me that there wasn't any great danger to worry about. Still, I was incredibly frustrated.

Actually, he was totally unbearable.

Well, it was January already, and spring training was right around the corner, in February. And I was gaining my weight back and building my strength – and then suddenly, I'm back to square one. So, yeah, Charisse is probably right about that.

But once again, Darryl overcame all the odds. He didn't let it set him back. Four or five days after that second surgery he was back at the gym, lifting weights again – with a row of staples holding his stomach together. I was furious, but I couldn't make him stop. Dr. Ihde told him, "Be careful. Give it a couple weeks' rest," but she couldn't stop him either. "Well," she gave in, "at least don't do any abdominal workouts." He tried to tell me he wouldn't do anything that stretched his stomach, but I knew better than to buy that. "How are you going to do upper-body workouts without stretching?" I asked him. But he just kept going to the gym. He was determined to get back to baseball so that he could take care of his family.

The only positive thing about that second operation was that it gave the doctors a chance to see how the first surgery had healed. Everything looked fine, with no signs of a recurring tumor. So when the incision Dr. Ihde had made healed enough so that she could take out Darryl's second set of staples, we felt like this time we were really out of the woods.

Now it was up to Nana's cooking to get Darryl back up to his playing weight.

Nana stayed at our house, and we ate potatoes. The doctors said potatoes would help me put on weight, and by the time Nana was done, I'd learned as much about potatoes from her as Forrest Gump learned from his friend "Bubba" about shrimp. I steered clear of the stuff I used to eat. No more Wendy's or Burger King. Just lots of fruit and vegetables – broccoli, yams, greens – and grilled or baked chicken, nothing fried. Normally in the off-season I avoid chicken like the plague, since when I'm on the road with the team it's something you see every night on hotel menus. But now I was eating a lot of chicken, because that's what the doctor ordered. And potatoes…

By the time we left for Tampa on Saturday, February 13, 1999, I weighed 235 pounds – twenty pounds over my normal playing weight.

Game Face

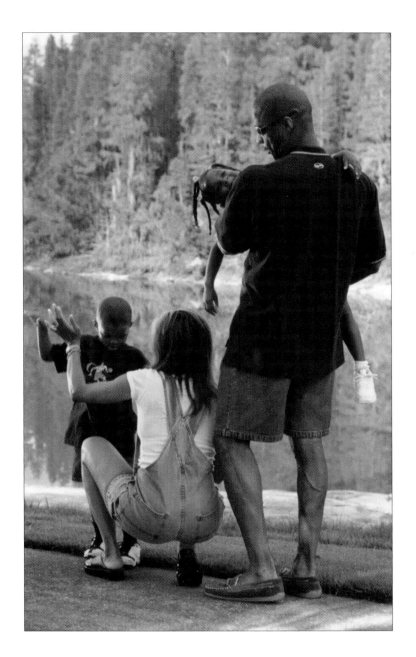

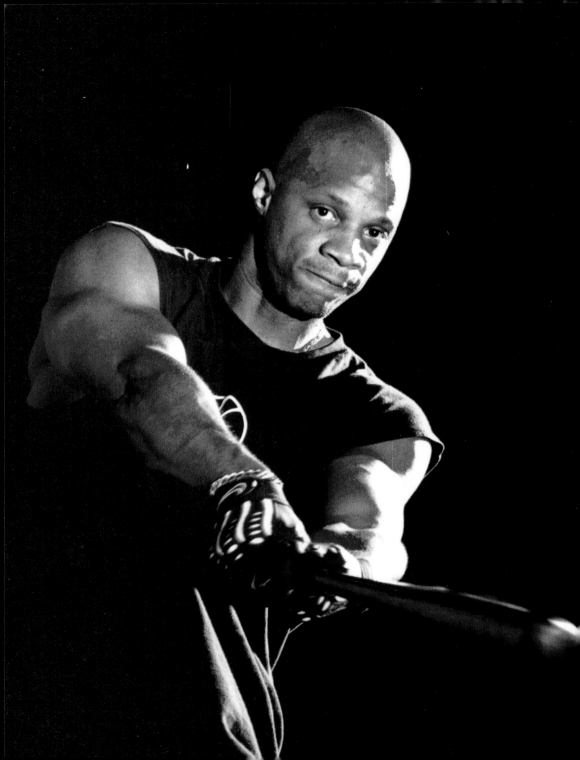

CHAPTER IX

CLEARING THE WALL

"Whenever anyone asked how I was feeling,
I would say without hesitation, 'Oh, I'm feeling fine.'"

"By four or five in the morning the media was there,
camped outside my house like a circus,
and I was growing desperate."

All through the off-season in California, I'd been telling my-self, "You're going to play again. Stay focused, and you'll be in the starting lineup on opening day." I was bound and determined not to let anything stop me from that goal. That's a trait I've always had: once I make up my mind about something, you can forget trying to change it.

So when Charisse, the kids, and I got down to Tampa, we focused our energy on getting set up and ready to roll so that I'd be ready to hit the field and prove to the team I was in playing shape. Once we were settled in we got my chemotherapy schedule lined up. I spent time at the Yankees' Legends Field minor league complex, putting in preliminary training work. Then on February 23 spring training began.

I hadn't seen most of my teammates since the victory parade after the World Series. Only a few months had passed since that day in New York, but I'd been through so much in that short stretch of time that it seemed years had gone by. Back then, we'd had no sure-fire guarantee that I'd make it through the winter, let alone be back for spring training.

Cancer is a frightening thing to have to face. Like I've said before, it forces you to reevaluate the things you think are important. At the same time, it reinforces your awareness of the things you enjoy most, and for me there's never been a question that one of those things is baseball. So it was a great feeling for me to meet up with the other guys at Legends Field and be back out on the diamond, even though deep down inside I knew I wasn't fully up to the demands of training quite yet.

The pre-season got underway, and I did my best to show my stuff in left field and at the plate while sticking to my weekly chemo schedule. I felt good about the way I was playing and confident in my hitting; it was a relief to know I could still punch a ball deep over the wall. The only thing troubling me was that no one would give me a definite answer about my status with the team. We'd worked out the contract – that was no longer a problem – but now I couldn't seem to get a straight answer from anyone about whether I'd be putting on my Yankee road grays when the team played the A's in Oakland to kick off the regular season. Even though my motto is "one day at a time," it made me antsy not to know what was up.

Still, so many people were rooting for me, wanting to see me make it back, that I had to keep giving my best effort. My family was behind me, and by that I don't just mean my wife and kids, but also my "cancer family," the people who knew what I was fighting through and wanted to see me succeed. Here's one letter that touched me and encouraged me to keep going, and I was needing all the encouragement I could get.

March 11, 1999

Dear Mr. Strawberry,

I hope this letter will actually find its way to you.

My name is Emily Voorhees. I was your next-door neighbor in the McKeen Pavilion of Columbia-Presbyterian Hospital; we passed each other on slow walks around the ward, IV stands in hand, but I don't think I ever introduced myself to you. I did, however, get to know your bodyguards – they called me "Smiley" and made me do just that each time I passed by. (They were especially helpful one night when, in the midst of what I assume was post-anesthesia daze, I got up from my bed, unassisted for the first time, and left my room convinced that I had to meet my family for dinner. The man sitting outside your door – I have forgotten his name – was kind enough to remind me of the reality of the situation. "Hey, Smiley, what are you doing up? It's 3:30 in the morning. Go back to sleep." I felt silly and confused, but instantly safe.) I left the hospital a couple of days before you did. I watched your press conference in the hospital from my hotel room when you left – so relieved to see you smiling, if only for the media's sake.

I was at Columbia-Presbyterian for brain surgery – they removed a peach-size tumor from the ventricle of my brain. I returned home to New Mexico where I had to have two more surgeries before returning to Middlebury College in Vermont at the beginning of January. It started snowing last night (as it does often in these parts) right as I turned on the TV and heard that you had a hit in your exhibition game against the Red Sox – congratulations! I was so happy to hear that. So happy. Even though I do not know you personally, I did feel a strange surge of personal excitement when I saw you on the 10:00 news – a huge victory for you after all you have been through. You are an inspiration to me, Mr. Strawberry, and a reminder not to waste a second, nor to be afraid to squeeze as much out of the time we have been given...

I hope this letter finds you because, most importantly, I want you to know how happy I was and, simply put, how *proud* I was when I heard about your game yesterday. It was an inspiration to me. I can understand that the past few months have not been remotely easy, but from one graduate of McKeen to another, I want to personally wish you the best. I am perhaps not your craziest fan, but I am an honest one.

Thank you and good luck to you and your family. God bless.

Emily Voorhees

Is he eating right? Are his bowel movements regular? Does he have diarrhea? How's his weight? Is he fatigued? Are there any more problems with scar tissue? Those were the questions that concerned me most during the off-season. Both Darryl and I measured his progress by physical indications, wanting to be sure everything was functioning properly and that he was gaining his strength again. We knew that those were the things the Yankee coaches and trainers would be concerned about when it came time to evaluate Darryl's ability to perform on the field. So we focused on making sure his body was recovering, on the physical side of his health.

Throughout much of the off-season, Darryl's contract was still in limbo. The thought that all his work to get back into shape might be in vain lurked at the back of our minds and created another element of stress. It was almost as if it never occurred to either of us to think how the pressures of battling cancer and the side effects of chemotherapy might be affecting him emotionally.

I don't think anyone from the team expected Darryl to show up for spring training in such good shape. Aside from Gene Monahan, the head trainer, who'd been out to California to check on Darryl back in December 1998, no one from the Yankees had seen him since his surgery in New York.

During spring training I think Darryl didn't talk about how he really felt because he was afraid he would be penalized for it. One time he admitted to being tired after chemo, and they took him out of the lineup for that night's game. He wanted so badly to play, to prove to himself and everyone else that he could contribute, and he didn't want to jeopardize his chances. If he had really come out and said how he was feeling mentally, he might have been penalized more. At least that's how I feel about it.

When the team flew to California for the final road trip of the pre-season, an Easter Weekend series with the Dodgers, Darryl went with them. He knew he'd have to return to Tampa to complete his chemotherapy, but he arranged with Joe Torre (he's the Yankees' manager) that he could stay with the team for this trip. I flew with the kids to Los Angeles, too, to be there with him, and we stayed at our house.

Darryl didn't seem himself that weekend. I could tell the stress was really getting to him. He wanted so badly to make the team, I think he would have quit chemo then and there if they would have let him. He and I decided it would be best for me to take the kids to New Jersey, so they could settle in by the time Darryl came up from Tampa. So on Easter Sunday I left with them on a flight to New York.

Monday, April 5, 1999. The Yankees played their first game of the season. But instead of sitting in the visitors' dugout, I found myself sitting in a plane, on a flight back to Tampa. I had to swallow hard and try to make the best of it. There was still plenty of time, I told myself.

The Yanks lost that first game, 5–3.

That weekend, the team played a three-game series against Detroit at Yankee Stadium, the first home stand of the year (Yankees 3, Tigers 0). I flew up to New York to participate in the "Welcome Home" dinner Thursday night at the downtown Sheraton. I sat there and signed autographs for the fans with the rest of the guys.

At the game on Sunday we were presented with our World Series rings, and I joined my teammates in remembering our fairy-tale championship season. I now had three pieces of diamond-studded hardware to my name, but knowing that after the game I would be returning to Florida instead of to the locker room made me feel a bit withdrawn from the excitement.

I wish I could say that when I got back to Tampa I put on my spikes and went to work with a smile so cheery it infected all the personnel at the training complex, leaving them with no choice but to recommend I get my butt up to New York on the next available flight. But that's not how it happened.

From the start, back when I first went in for surgery on my colon, my doctors warned me that sooner or later every cancer patient hits a wall. At some point, they said, I'd reach a point where I would feel unable to go on. "Don't be surprised," they said. "It's the same for everyone."

Like Charisse said, though, our focus was on my physical wellbeing. And in that way I tried to fool myself. I told myself I've always been strong, I've always pulled through. I wasn't going to let cancer get the better of me, and I promised myself I'd fight through it – especially after my second surgery in January, when I began to feel the chemo wearing me down. It took a toll on my energy level. Sometimes I felt lightheaded, dizzy. Other times, I got angry or was moody and didn't want to talk about anything. Everyone around me was moving forward, but I felt myself standing still. Sometimes it felt like I was going backward, getting farther from the goal I wanted to reach. But whenever anyone asked how I was feeling, I would say without hesitation, "Oh, I'm feeling fine."

Maybe I'm stubborn, or just naïve, but I tuned out the doctors' warnings about "hitting walls" and stuff like that. I refused to think about the possibility of side effects from the chemo influencing me in any way. The voice inside my head kept reminding me, "You're going to have to come back and prove that you can play left field again. You're going to have to come back and prove a point..."

It's been an uphill struggle for Darryl all the way. That's how it's always been for him. He's faced drug and alcohol issues, legal problems, back surgery that robbed him of playing time in Los Angeles, and a knee operation that took away his 1997 season in New York. One hurdle after another.

In 1998 he finally gets his chance to be a positive force in the lineup, hitting home runs and helping the team win. And then: cancer. "God, what else?" was all I could say...

I was alone in Tampa. My family wasn't with me. My teammates weren't around me. Thoughts of recurring cancer still gnawed at me, and the poisons of chemotherapy still had to be reckoned with each week. I tried to stay positive, to concentrate on my workouts and practice sessions, but each day it became harder to keep focused.

I'd get home in the afternoon and sleep like crazy. Then I'd wake up with mad headaches, and be angry at the world...

I see myself: I'm not playing, and I don't know when I'll be playing. But I have to go back to the park each morning and go through my routine again. And every day the pressure builds higher...

Where was my faith in all of this? I was hanging on, but just barely. Back in California, I could count on the encouragement of people close to us, our friends who pray for us every day and stand alongside us through everything we go through, and I had the Spiritual 12-Step program to help me. Now, though, I was on my own. My depression grew to the point where I started talking outside of myself. I knew the voice well, but it wasn't one I ever thought I'd hear again: it was the voice of the old Darryl, the Darryl that knew only one solution to any problem.

I just couldn't stop myself. For the first time in over four years, I took a drink.

And that's when I hit my wall.

It wasn't much after eleven o'clock in the evening on Wednesday, April 14, when the phone rang. Eric Grossman was on the line. "Charisse, I have bad news," were his first words. He sounded frantic, hurt. I went numb. Something had happened to Darryl, I was certain. "What?" I asked. "What's going on?" I didn't know what to expect. I sure didn't expect to listen to Eric telling me Darryl had been arrested in downtown Tampa and charged with soliciting prostitution (from an undercover cop, as it turned out) and carrying cocaine in his wallet. I didn't want to believe what I was hearing. "What?" I kept saying.

Eric did his best to tell me the details as he understood them. The police had called the Yankees, and someone from the front office had called him. Darryl had been taken to a jail, he told me, but he'd be out on bail in an hour or so.

By the time I got off the phone I was shaking. I tried to think, but the shock wouldn't go away. The kids were asleep. I was the only one awake in the house; Nana had already left a few days earlier. I called my girlfriend Patti, and she said she'd come right over. Then I called a few other people: my dad, the Leonards, and Josh. I also called Ron Dock, the Yankees' intervention coordinator down in Tampa, a man who understands recovery from his own experience. He went straight over to the jail to be with Darryl.

My girlfriend pulled in, and she stayed with me all night. At first I had this wild idea that maybe the whole thing was some weird mistake. It just didn't sound like Darryl to me — at least not the Darryl I was used to. Maybe, I told myself, just maybe the media won't catch wind of this and it'll all blow over. But I kept the TV tuned to ESPN, just in case. Of course it didn't take long for the story to break. Once it hit, I switched off the TV. I didn't want to sit through whatever they had to say. I turned out all the lights in the house, because I knew it would only be a matter of minutes before the media was at the doorstep.

Even if I'd been able to, there was no way I could have slept that night. The phone rang nonstop. Sometime in the early morning I had a chance to talk to Darryl.

"Are you all right?" I asked him.

"I'm hurting," he said.

"I'll be there in the morning."

"Okay."

"We'll deal with it then."

That's about all either of us managed.

By four or five in the morning the media was there, camped outside my house like a circus, and I was growing desperate. There was no way I was talking to them. They weren't looking for Darryl. They were looking for me, and I wasn't going to have my picture or my kids' splashed on the front page with some catchy line about Darryl's downfall.

I had booked a commercial morning flight out of Newark, and I was dreading the thought of having to go through the airport with the kids. Then at the last minute a friend rang the house and offered to fly us down to Tampa in a private aircraft. I gratefully accepted, and in my heart I said a silent prayer of thanks. At a time when I was feeling very alone, it was so good to know we still had friends who would stick with us regardless of what was happening.

I threw some things in a suitcase, not knowing how long we'd be gone, and Patti helped me get the kids fed and dressed. Then we got into the SUV in our garage and, since there were still a few reporters milling around on the street, my kids and I sat on the floor of the truck until Patti got us out of our neighborhood. Jordan and Jade had no idea what was going on. I told them we were going to play a game and try to hide from the bad Power Rangers. They bought into it and had a great time. I'm sure they were thinking, Wow, this is great! Mommy's in the back with us on the floor. Usually she's telling us to sit down and stay in our car seats... I, on the other hand, was in a whirlwind, or maybe more like a nightmare. I wanted to know when I was going to wake up.

My one source of comfort was that right from the moment Eric called me, I never believed Darryl had actually been trying to solicit sex. I felt confident enough in our relationship not to worry about that. From what I knew about recovery and addictions, I realized something else was at the root of what had happened. Darryl had been trying to fight two diseases at once – cancer and alcoholism – and it seemed he'd been losing to the second one. The night of his arrest, he'd been thinking about taking another step backward.

By noon Thursday, the kids and I were in the air, flying to Tampa. And then, there I was, facing Darryl.

"I'm sorry." What are those words supposed to mean after you've said them a thousand times? How can you expect anyone to believe you mean them, and even if they give you the benefit of the doubt, so what? – what does "sorry" change? And why is it always the people you're the closest to, whom you end up hurting the most?

Those were the kinds of questions going through my head as I waited for Charisse to arrive. I knew I didn't have any answers, at least none that could make anything right. I wished I did.

This much I know: I know that I have a wife who is the most special gift God has given me. Even in my darkest moments, when I am to blame for her anger and tears, she refuses to judge me.

I fall on my face and the world says, "Oh, look at him. He's messed up, and just when everyone was doing so much for him." But Charisse understands the stress and strain I battle each day, both as a recovering addict and alcoholic and as a cancer victim. She knows that just because I've turned my life over to God, it doesn't mean things get easier. She doesn't accept my faults or make excuses for me, but neither does she run when trouble comes my way. And each day, believe me, I thank God for her.

Charisse knows me so well. Like she says, from the first news of my arrest she grasped that solicitation wasn't the issue. She just knew that wasn't me. When that undercover Tampa officer suggested I meet her in a motel parking lot, I didn't take her seriously. That's why I was already two blocks past it when the officers backing her up pulled me over on Kennedy Boulevard.

I never intended to follow through. That helped me behave like a gentleman during my arrest and arraignment. But it was Charisse's understanding and strength that would end up carrying me through the hearings and court appearances still ahead.

Of course I was upset when I got to Tampa, and I let Darryl know it. He felt terrible about what had happened and apologized many times. We shared a lot of tears together. Darryl is a good person. He has a good heart. It wasn't like he was flippant about it or anything, and I knew we'd work through everything together.

Back when Darryl and I met and started dating, we both believed strongly that God brought us together for a reason. Since then, we've been through a lot, and there have been times when Darryl has asked me, "Do you ever wish you'd never married me?" Each time, I've given him the same answer: "No. God put me in your life. He wanted me to marry you, so of course there's a reason."

I believe that, and I know Darryl does too. Even back at the very beginning of our relationship, it seemed clear to both of us that God was bringing us together for a reason. I think God knew – of course he knew – all the things that we were going to go through.

Each of us has things we're afraid of. I'm always afraid of failing. I know I'm only human and that mistakes are part of life, but just knowing that isn't enough to make my fear of failure go away.

The fear of letting God down – that's a different kind of fear than, say, letting down your boss or your colleagues or something like that. I know there have been many times when I've let God down, and nothing saddens me more. I don't think anyone ever deliberately sets out to make mistakes, but for some reason they still happen. And when I make mistakes, I'm very ashamed. I'm ashamed, because it truly hurts knowing how good God is to me and how he looks out for me. At the same time, though, I believe each time any of us makes a mistake, we are faced with a choice: do we give up and quit, or do we try to learn from it and grow stronger as a result? If there's one thing I know, it's that God never quits. So what right do I have to quit on him?

To play professional baseball demands hard work. Even if it's what you enjoy doing most, you still have to be completely dedicated to it; otherwise, you're not going to be in shape either physically or mentally to be able to perform. It's a daily thing, and it doesn't end when the season's over and everyone goes home. During the off-season, just like during the regular season, you've got to maintain fitness: lift weights, ride exercise bikes, stretch, run, sweat. You've got to make sure you're eating right and getting proper rest. If you want to be a competitor, those are the things you worry about and focus on.

And you just can't decide you're going to slacken off for a day or two. If you do, you'll pay for it in ways you don't expect. Before you know it, you lose your work habits, and once you've lost those, you fall off track quickly. You start going backward. All your hard work amounts to nothing unless you stick with it, every day.

After Darryl's arrest, he picked himself right back up and got back on track. Josh flew in from California to support us, putting his life on hold to be there when we needed him most. Together, he and Darryl started working a program, attending two meetings every day.

Darryl knows that if he loses his sobriety and goes back to his old ways, he loses everything else. No more baseball. No family, most likely. If he doesn't have his sobriety, he doesn't have Darryl. If he didn't know these things before, he sure knows them now. That helps keep him on track, and gives me a lot of courage for the future.

More than ever before, I now understand that what it takes to be a winning ball player is no different from what it takes to win when you're in recovery. There's a parallel between the two. To recover from addiction demands spiritual dedication. Just like in normal life, if your spirit isn't being fed a healthy diet every day, you get weak and sick. And if you don't do spiritual workouts, you lose your strength.

That's where meditation and prayer come in. It's funny how prayer can turn things around. When I was arrested in Tampa, I felt like the things I'd worked to maintain over the recent years — my sobriety, my health, my marriage — might suddenly be ruined. The irony is that not long before I had been asked by an author friend of mine, Christoph Arnold, to write a foreword for a book he was writing on the meaning and power of prayer. Christoph lost his mother to cancer and has undergone surgery for tumors himself. He knows the importance of prayer for anyone facing serious illness, which is why he asked me to contribute. In the fore-word to his book *Cries from the Heart*, I wrote that "the bedrock of my faith is prayer." At the time, I had no idea my own words would be put to the test so soon. But with Charisse by my side, I found that they hold true — that when you hang on to faith and turn your mind back to God, asking him to take control, then he'll show you the way around any roadblock.

Mostly these days my prayers consist of saying "thank you" to God. I know I have every reason to be thankful, and I want to re-mind myself of that as each day begins: "Thank you that I'm alive… Thank you for my family, for my wife… Thank you for wak-ing me up to see a new day… Thank you for staying with me, every step of my life – even when I didn't know you were there…"

I think thankfulness is so important. Strange as it sounds, I'm now able to look back on my arrest in April and actually give thanks for it. I realize that even though it cost me a lot of pain and humiliation, God used that moment to bring me up short. I could have gone back to being a drinker and user. Instead, I got ar-rested, and that jolted me back to my senses.

At one time, I never thought much about my life, about the meaning of any of us being here. It's something else that cancer has helped me to see. Now I realize there are no guarantees. On any given day, you can drop dead. That makes me thankful, and I want God to know that I am. What's important to me now is not being a baseball player or anything like that. It's being able to see each day as a chance to start life over, and not to waste time.

No matter what I'm doing during the day, I can be talking to God in my heart. I want to remember that as I continue my comeback to baseball. I look forward to hitting more home runs and being a force on the field. In baseball and in life, my goals amount to the same thing. Through it all, I know that if I truly seek for God's will in my life, then I'm going to find it. That's a promise.

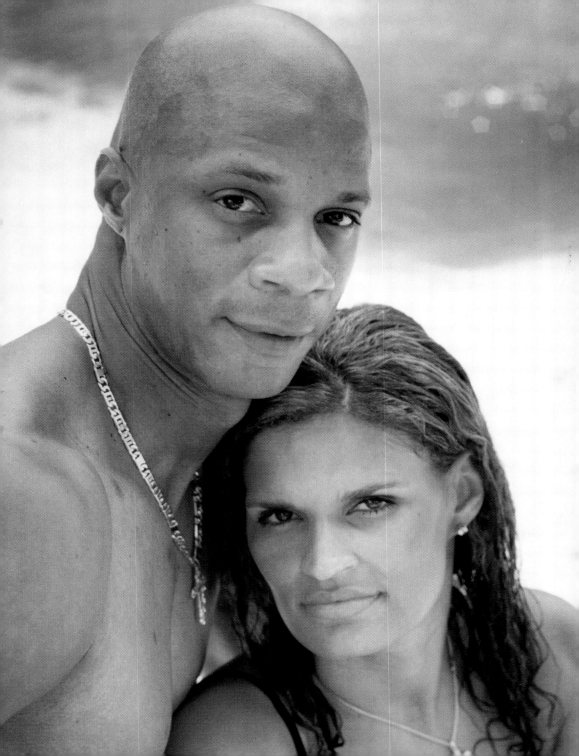

BEYOND BASEBALL

Our pastor at St. Stephen, E. Wilbert McCall, likes to remind us, "You're either in a storm, coming out of a storm, or heading into a new storm." That means there are two times when you're not in a storm: when you're coming out of one, and when you're getting ready for the next one – and they amount to the same thing.

Over the last years this thought has kept returning to me. The way I see it, this is the point: Try not to get lost in whatever storm you're dealing with. Focus on something beyond it, and keep moving forward. Accept the fact that life is going to be a constant battle; otherwise, you'll always be frustrated and you'll never find peace.

I've always believed that in the end, if we stand by each other and put our trust in God to see us through, everything will work out for the good.

I think both Darryl and I are pretty honest about things, or at least we try to be. We have our days, good and bad. We know we're not special, not any different from anyone else.

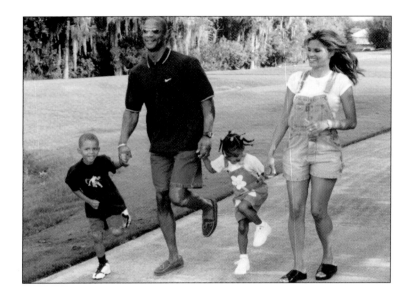

Regardless of what the media says or what people choose to think, we're pretty normal.

The important thing for anyone, I think, is to remember that one day each of us has to face God on our own. That's why it's pointless to waste energy on judging other people. Deal with your own problems. If you need a program, find a program and work it. We've each got to start with ourselves, and then we'll do a much better job of helping others.

Look around. There are doctors and lawyers and business executives all going through the same thing – there's no level of society that isn't affected in some way by drugs or alcohol – but they can't speak about these issues. Maybe, though, hearing from someone like Darryl, someone whose dirty laundry has been put through the spin cycle by the media, would be a help to them somewhere down the line.

In the past, we've had chances to speak out about our battle with the "family disease," and we'll welcome more opportunities in the future. Darryl and I both hope we can continue to bring something positive to people of all ages by speaking honestly to them about our own failings and the issues we deal with, and by being open with them about the problems they face. That's what it boils down to – being honest and speaking about difficult things. At least that's where it has to start. From there, we can all work together to break the cycle for our children's sake.

In talking about how this book should end, Charisse and I asked ourselves, "What do we want people to take away with them when they're done with it?" My hope is that the things we've talked about, the stories we've shared – both the happy memories and the ones we'd rather forget – will be an encouragement to others, particularly readers suffering from substance abuse.

Here's my advice: I know what it's like to be humiliated because of addictions. I know what it's like to be afraid. But you've got to overcome fear. Find someone to help you, a friend you can trust. Don't be afraid to step up and acknowledge your problems. Don't be afraid to admit that there are serious issues your family needs to face. Because if you don't, your kids are going to fall into the same pattern one day.

Thankfully, not every family has to battle the demons of addiction, but there are always forces trying to tear families apart, looking for a chance to wreck lives. I can witness to their power. At the same time, though, I can witness to the power of God, which is even stronger. It's like a mighty hand, reaching down to grab hold of you. Even when you think you're finished, when you're ready to give up, it's still there. All you have to do is take that hand – and then let go of everything else. "Let go and let God." And somehow, when the storm has passed, you'll find yourself back on your feet again, ready to go on. One day at a time.

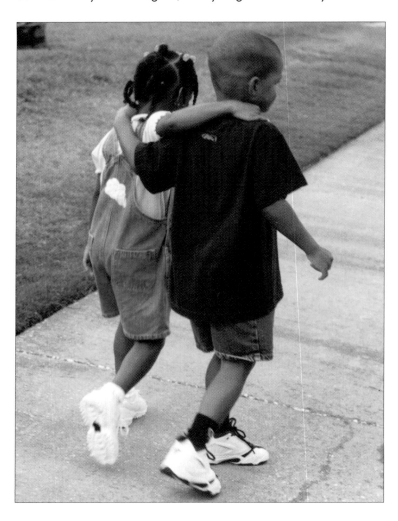

ACKNOWLEDGMENTS

This book grew out of many conversations – between the two of us, with our friends, and with the team at The Plough Publishing House. We thank all those who assisted us throughout the writing process and helped bring this book into being.

Our thanks, too, to George Steinbrenner and the entire New York Yankees organization. You have stood by us through some of the best, and some of the worst, chapters of our lives. Without you, this book might never have been written. Because of you, we look forward to "chapters" still to come.

Finally, our thanks to the many baseball fans whose prayers and goodwill bring so much encouragement to us. You know who you are, and we thank you.

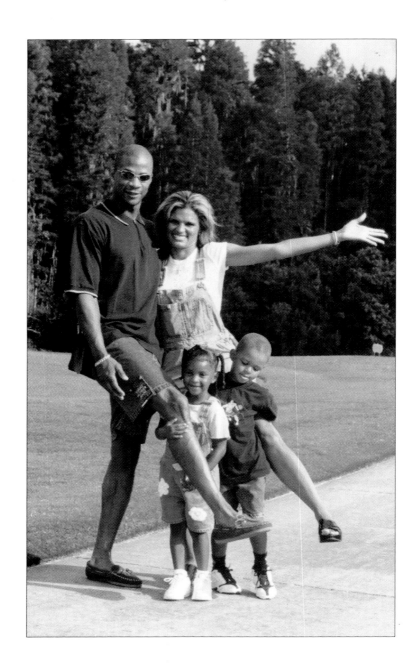